O. Kleinsasser

Microlaryngoscopy and Endolaryngeal Microsurgery

Third edition

Microlaryngoscopy and Endolaryngeal Microsurgery

Technique and Typical Findings

Oskar Kleinsasser, M.D.

Professor of Medicine
Head, Division of Otorhinolaryngology
Philipps-University Marburg Medical Clinic
Marburg, Germany

Translated by
P. M. Stell Ch. M. FRCS, A.I.L.
Professor of Oto-Rhino-Laryngology
Head, University Department of
Oto-Rhino-Laryngology
Royal Liverpool Hospital
Liverpool, England

Third, completely revised edition

HANLEY & BELFUS, INC./Philadelphia
MOSBY – YEAR BOOK, INC./St. Louis • Baltimore • Boston • Chicago • London
Philadelphia • Sydney • Toronto

Publisher: HANLEY & BELFUS, INC.
210 S. 13th Street
Philadelphia, PA 19107

North American and worldwide sales and distribution:
THE C.V.MOSBY COMPANY
11830 Westline Industrial Drive
St. Louis, MO 63146

In Canada: THE C.V.MOSBY COMPANY
5240 Finch Avenue East
Unit 1
Scarborough, Ontario M1S 4P2

Authorized translation of the third German language edition

Title of the original edition:
Mikrolaryngoskopie und endolaryngeale Mikrochirurgie

Microlaryngoscopy and Endolaryngeal Microsurgery

ISBN I-56053-006-5

 Library of Congress Catalog card number 91-68451

Last digit is the print number: 9 8 7 6 5 4 3 2 1

Dedicated to my wife

Foreword to the Third Edition

Thirty years have passed since the very first beginnings of microlaryngoscopy and microsurgery. Both techniques are now standard methods in laryngology. With the help of microlaryngoscopy we learned on the one hand how to detect the premalignant lesions and very early stages of laryngeal cancer as well as a broad spectrum of benign diseases, and on the other hand how to differentiate them from each other. Endolaryngeal microsurgery enables us to resect a certain number of smaller cancers and benign lesions for the purpose of restitution of the patient's voice.

The first edition of this book was published in 1968, and the second followed in 1976. In the meantime, the techniques dealt with were subject to further sophisticated development. Therefore, the text of the present third edition has been completely rewritten and expanded. As for the color figures, some of the most expressive ones were reused from the first two editions. A great number of photographs were replaced by others that are more exact from a technical point of view. We supplied many new figures, including representations of less common diseases, thus almost doubling the number of illustrations compared to previous editions.

I would like to thank my colleagues and my fellow surgeons at the University Clinic of Otorhinolaryngology at Marburg for their always helpful assistance as well as for providing several photographs reproduced in this edition.

Mr. Karl Storz, M.D.h.c., and his colleagues helped me over the course of three decades in developing and continuously improving the instrumentation for microlaryngoscopy and endolaryngeal microsurgery.

I also wish to express my thanks to Prof. Philip M. Stell Ch.M., F.R.C.S., Professor of Otorhinolaryngology, University of Liverpool, for his expert and precise translation of the German text.

Mrs. Ingrid Wagner undertook the troublesome typing; Mrs. Monica Schüler had under her care the collection of photographs and assisted me in taking innumerable new pictures.

Once more I am grateful to Mr. D. Bergemann and Mr. Wulf Bertram M.D. for generously meeting my requests.

Marburg, autumn 1991

O. Kleinsasser

Contents

Introduction

I General Section

II Special Section

Introduction

This book is again divided into two main sections.

The first section provides a thorough description of the technique of endoscopic examination of the larynx and recording of the findings by photography and video tape. The instruments for microlaryngoscopy are described, the endolaryngeal operative techniques are presented, and the indications and contraindications for surgery, including pre- and postoperative procedures, are detailed. The author's experience with numerous courses has shown that this chapter needed more accurate and broader treatment than in previous editions. A historical review has been omitted because it was already published in the 2nd edition and has also been recently provided by Hans von Leden.[37] The 2nd edition of this book also comprises a thorough review of the modern literature[23] so that the only references included in this edition are those from more recent publications that are relevant to the present text. The second section is in the form of an atlas showing the most important microlaryngoscopic views of the numerous diseases of the larynx. This section, too, has been considerably expanded to include photographs of a wide range of unusual diseases of the larynx. As did Lehmann and his colleagues,[40] I have had to forgo publication of the corresponding histopathological appearances because of the very large number of illustrations. The text in the atlas part of the book has been deliberately kept to a minimum and is limited to the prevalence of the disease discussed, its incidence by age and sex, the pathogenesis and treatment of the individual disease, and its prognosis.

General Section

1. Examination of the Larynx

Modern laryngology has a wide range of diagnostic methods with which every laryngologist must be completely familiar. Microlaryngoscopy is an invasive procedure. It is usually the last step in the diagnostic work-up and is carried out immediately before the initiation of therapy.

Every examination of the larynx begins with **indirect laryngoscopy**, which allows a diagnosis to be made in up to 90% of cases provided that the examiner makes full use of the method. It is done after inducing mucosal anesthesia, if necessary.

Direct laryngoscopy using topical anesthesia and sedation is unappealing both to the patient and the surgeon; I only use it very occasionally, because it can be supplanted by other methods.

Indirect microlaryngoscopy (Figure 1) requires some skill on the part of the examiner and the cooperation of the patient to allow observation of the magnified view of the larynx obtained through the operating microscope. A large laryngeal mirror, a 30 mm objective on the operating microscope, and topical anesthesia facilitate the examination. However, increasing magnification reduces the depth of focus and makes focusing difficult. The advantage of this method is that it provides a binocular reflected image of the larynx in a way that is not possible with a head mirror, but the binocular effect is limited because the objective lenses of the operating microscope lie close together. However, this method does allow **microstroboscopy** to be achieved by coupling the operating microscope to a stroboscope.

The development of endoscopes with a rod-lens system and fiberglass transport of a cold light source has produced excellent examination instruments.[48] These laryngoscopes are termed loupe laryngoscopes in German-speaking countries[56] because the magnification is small, but in fact the optical system consists of several lenses rather than a singel loupe (Figure 2). Modern telescopic laryngoscopes have wide-angle objectives, producing an image that is sharp at the periphery and a depth of focus of practically nil to infinity. Some models have fixed focus, but the focus of others can be varied using a zoom, so that the magnification and the view can be altered simply. Telescopes of 90° and 70° allow examination not only of the pharynx and larynx but also of the nasopharynx if the instrument is rotated. A protective sleeve on the laryngoscope prevents contact of the front lens with saliva and also holds the uvula, the soft palate, and the base of the tongue away from the laryngoscope (Figure 2).

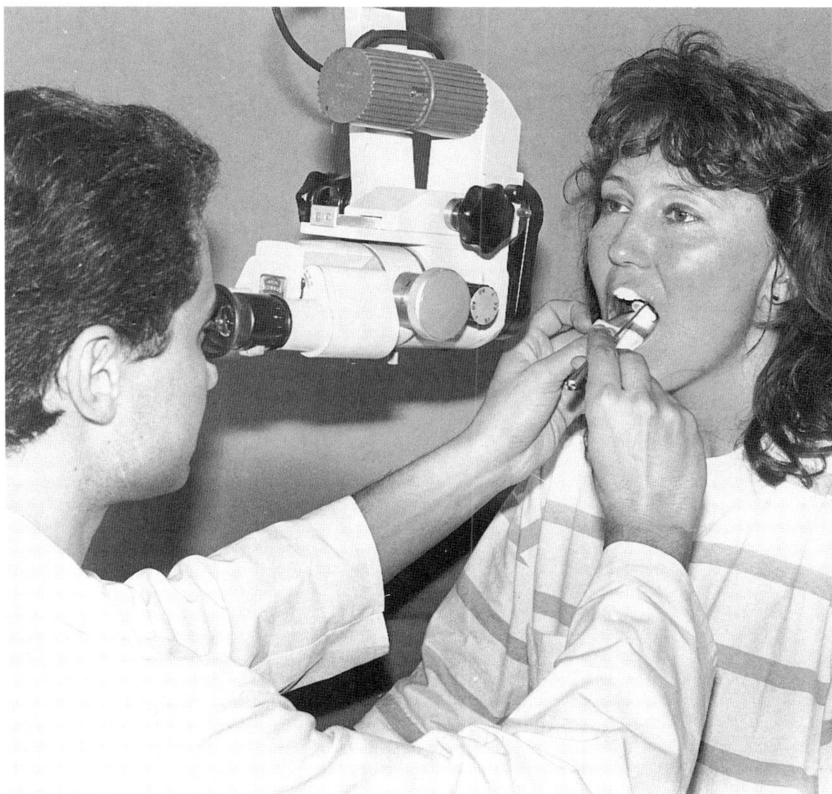

Fig. 1.

Indirect microlaryngoscopy showing the larynx illuminated by the operating microscope. The reflected image of the larynx is observed through the operating microscope at almost any desired magnification. An eyepiece with a focal length of 300 mm should be used to provide a satisfactory working distance. Microstroboscopy can be carried out by reflected stroboscopic light through the operating microscope.

The laryngeal telescope is now a routinely used instrument that allows accurate assessment of laryngeal disease. A beam splitter and a side-arm allow an observer to share in the examination (Figure 3). A video can be examined by the surgeon, by an observer, and also by the patient himself.[60]

The quality of the image provided by a **fiberoptic laryngoscope**[50] with a diameter of 3 or 4 mm has improved greatly in the last few years and may well now have reached the optimum that is technically possible (Figure 4). This instrument has already reached its limits of resolution, even with the finest fibers of the best quality, because the grid of the cross-section of the glass fibers interferes with vision, even at low magnification. Fiberoptic laryngoscopy requires practice, and anesthesia of the nasal and pharyngeal mucosa is needed. The method is particularly useful for unfavorable anatomical conditions such as a thick tongue base, an overhanging epiglottis, or laryngeal scars that render accurate inspection by any other means impossible. Fiberoptic laryngoscopy is also very useful for functional studies, because the end of the laryngoscope hangs in the pharynx and does not distort phonation. We also routinely use the fiberoptic laryngoscope for bronchoscopy in patients who have previously had a laryngectomy, and for retrograde laryngoscopy on patients with a tracheostomy. The disadvantages of fiberoptic laryngoscopy are the high cost and vulnerability of the instrument, and the laborious procedures for sterilization dictated by the fear of infection with AIDS. The instrument must be sterilized before every examination, therefore, a surgeon with a large practice needs several instruments.

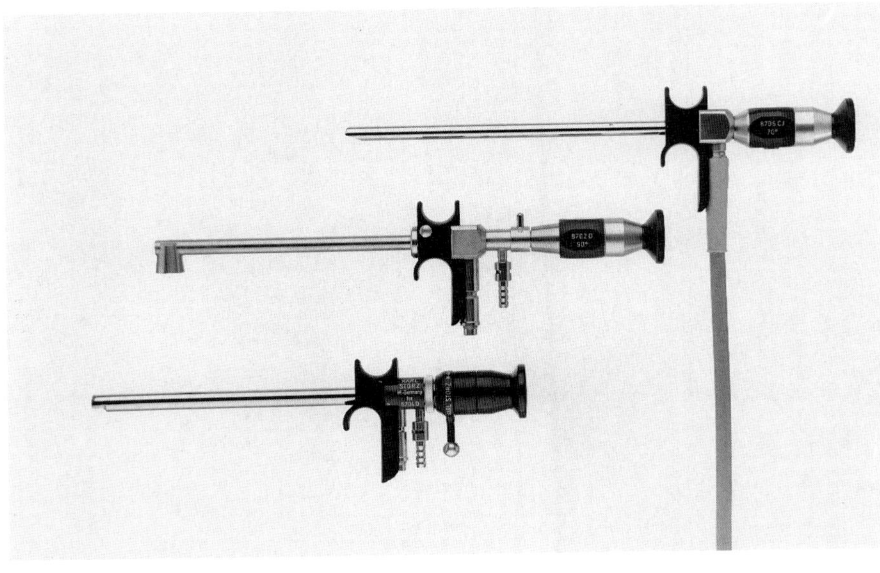

Fig. 2.

Telescopic laryngoscope with a right-angled lens, 70° lens, fixed focus, and variable focus. The protective hood prevents smearing of the eyepiece and pushes the uvula and the base of the tongue out of the field of vision.

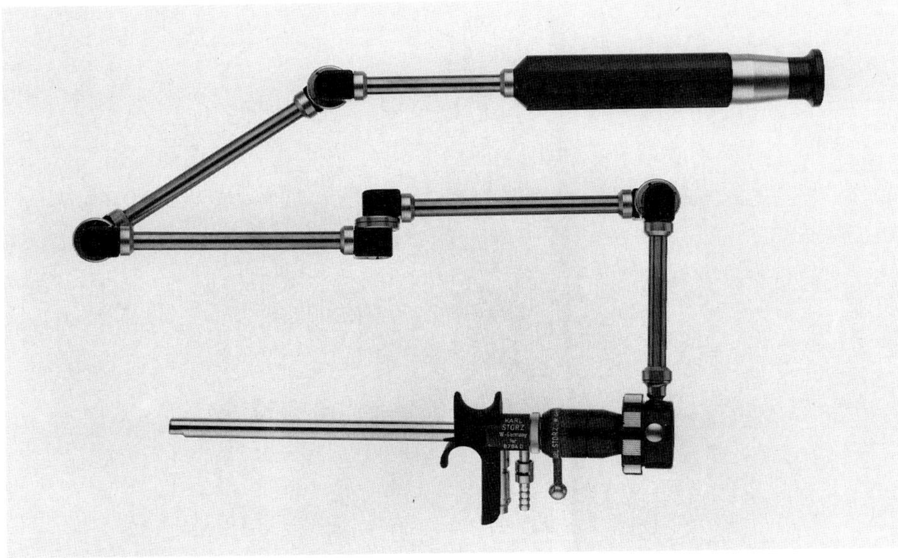

Fig. 3.

Telescopic laryngoscope with beam splitter and observation eyepiece.

An interesting future development may be the **chip endoscope.** The image is picked up by a microchip and electronically transmitted to a screen. At the moment the technique is not developed to the point where the chips, which should have a diameter of 3–4 mm and be carried on the thin flexible cable, can be introduced into the pharynx and larynx.

Every laryngologist should be able to carry out **stroboscopy.** The instrument has now been much simplified and is coupled with a telescope so that it can be used in the office (Figure 5). Stroboscopy provides important additional information, especially in vocal cord paralysis, small tumors, and especially for follow-up of vocal cord function.[21, 51]

Biopsies. These are nowadays almost always taken during microlaryngoscopy. Indirect laryngoscopic surgery is a dying art and indeed has never been taught or practiced in many countries. Biopsies taken by the indirect route with the help of a mirror are still indicated if microlaryngoscopy carries a high risk. Biopsies can also be taken from the larynx using a fiberoptic laryngoscope with a channel for instruments (Figure 6).

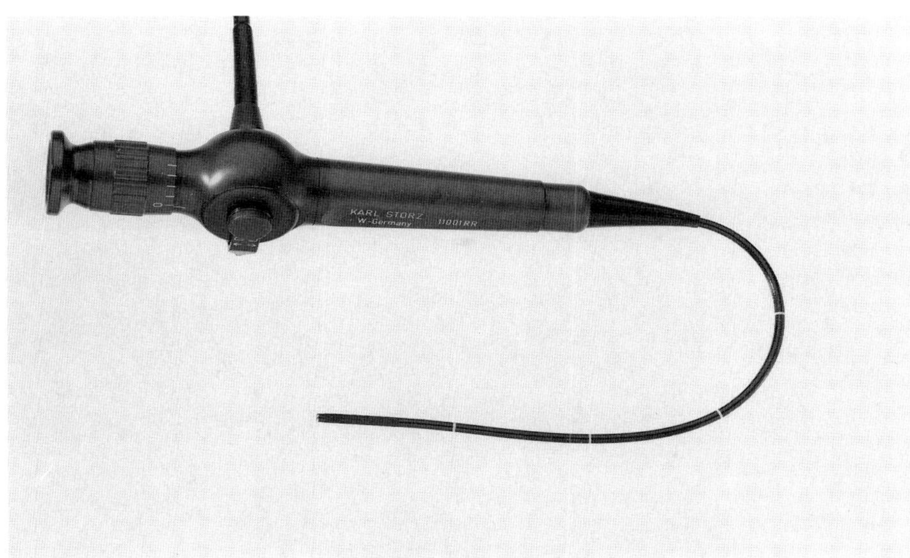

Fig. 4.

Fiberoptic laryngoscope for transnasal examination of the pharynx and larynx.

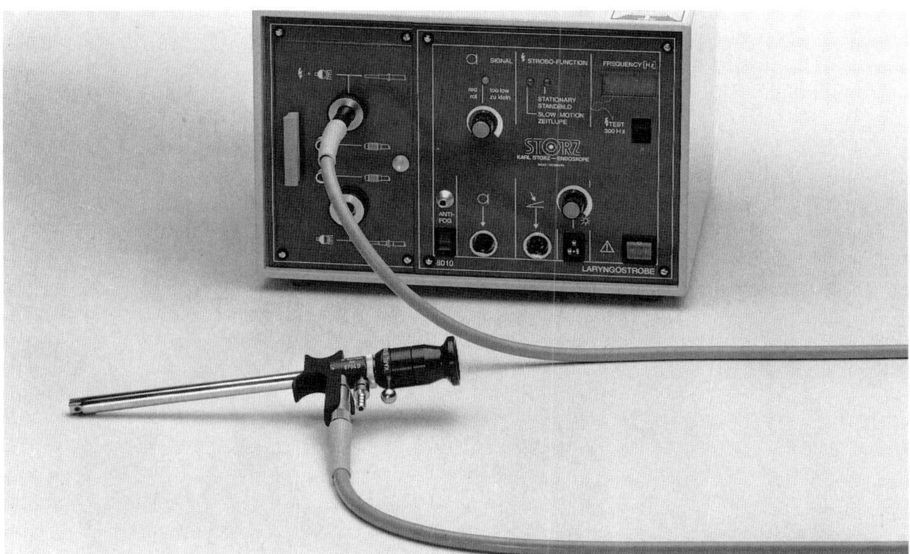

Fig. 5.

Stroboscope combined with a laryngoscopic telescope.

Nipping off of vocal cord polyps or nodules by the indirect route, even with the use of a fiberoptic laryngoscope, has now been abandoned. Even the most experienced surgeon cannot carry out the procedure as accurately by this route as by microlaryngoscopy.

Additional Investigations. A diagnosis is almost always achieved by endoscopy, and supplementary investigations such as conventional radiographs, tomography, CT scans, MRI scans, ultrasound, and electromyography to elucidate specific points are seldom needed. The questions to be answered include the depth of a tumor, its inferior extent, whether there is invasion of the laryngeal skeleton, and so forth.

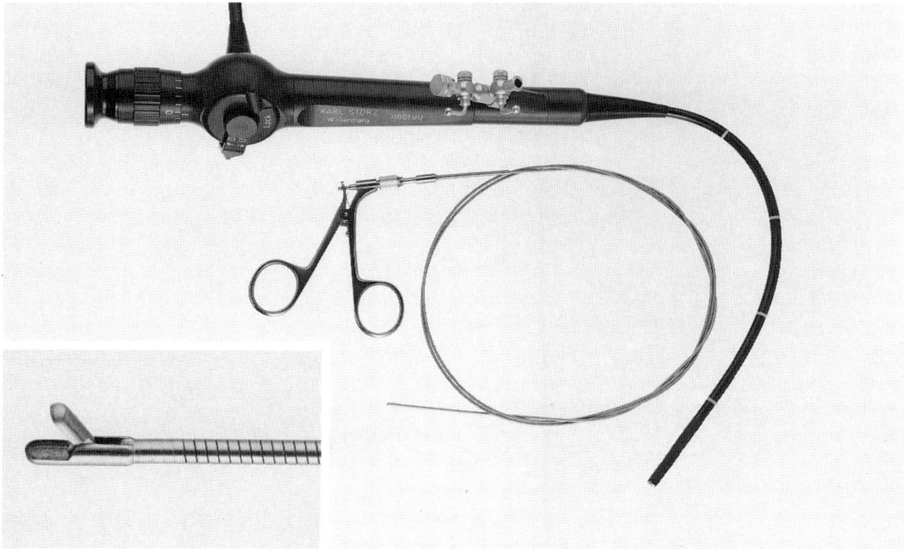

Fig. 6.

Fiberoptic laryngoscope with an instrument channel and double-cupped forceps for biopsy.

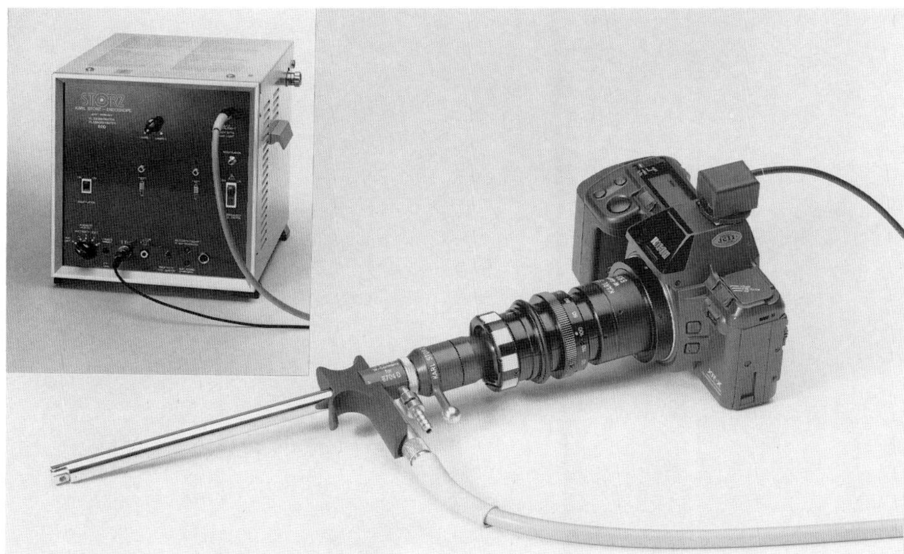

Fig. 7.

Laryngeal photography through the telescope. An electronically monitored flash light source is used with an autodynamic flash.

2. Photography and Video Recording

Photography of the larynx has a long history extending back to the last century.[23] The recent rapid developments in endoscopy, photography, and videorecording have now made it possible to take high quality views of the larynx more simply.

Photography Using the Telescope. Laryngeal telescopes with a 70° or 90° angle and with fixed focus or variable magnification are available. A monocular mirror-reflex camera with a zoom objective and a through-the-lens light meter have been adapted to the laryngeal telescope. The advantages include a spot meter instead of a integrated light meter and a clear glass focusing screen with a graticule for focusing. The light source is provided by an electronically controlled flash, and the light is transported by one or two glass-fiber cables. A cable release or foot switch and motorized film transport are advantageous (Figure 7).

The procedure requires some practice, mucosal anesthesia of the pharynx, the cooperation of the patient, and favorable anatomical conditions, but it provides sharp images filling the frame using daylight film. The camera and a laryngeal telescope together are somewhat heavy, cumbersome, and expensive when combined with a flash light-source.

Photography Using the Fiberoptic Laryngoscope. A beam splitter is used, and the camera and zoom objective are coupled to the second eyepiece, leaving one eyepiece free for focusing (Figure 8). The procedure demands mucosal anesthesia of the nose and pharynx and has the advantage that a good view of

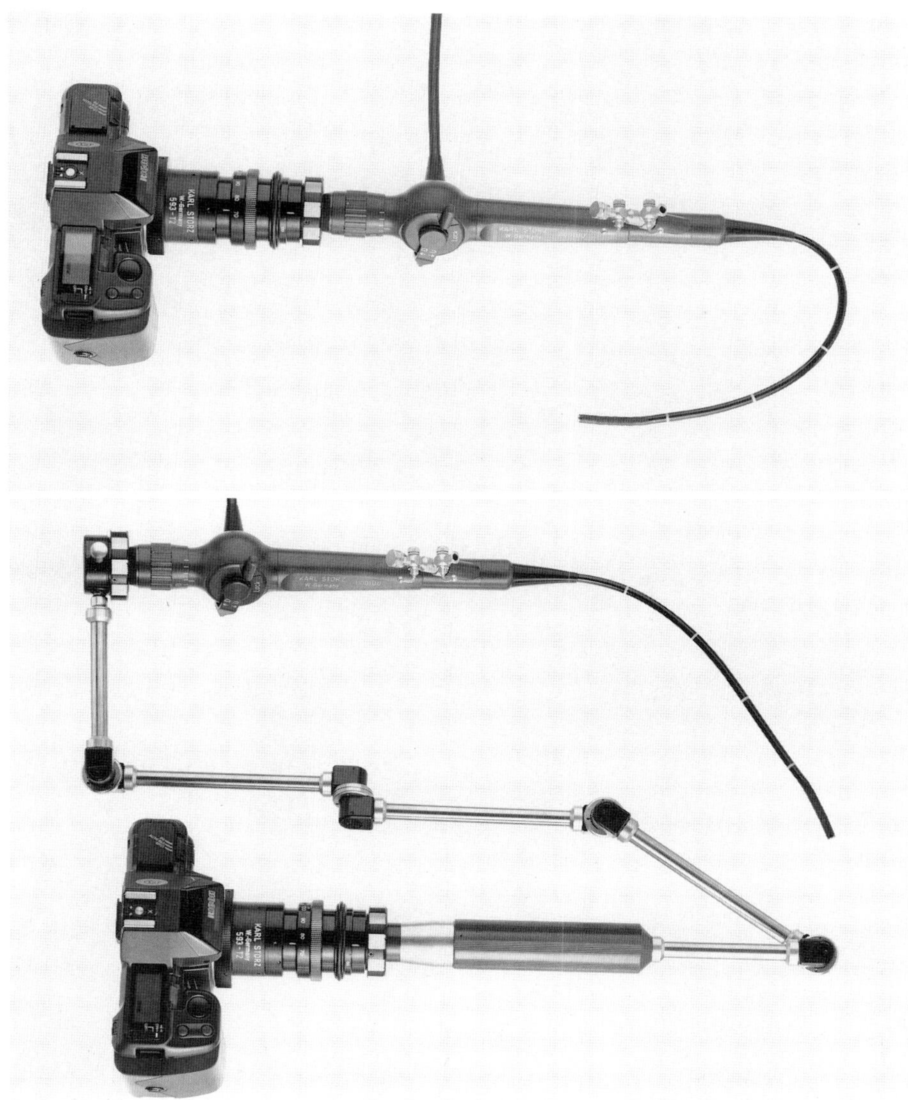

Fig. 8.

Laryngeal photography through the fiberoptic laryngoscope. The camera is fitted to the second eyepiece of the beam splitter, and illumination is provided by the flash light source shown in Figure 7.

conditions, without interfering with the function of the larynx. However, the quality of the photographs is not a good as that achieved through a rigid telescope; the picture does not fill the frame and enlargement produces interference by the fibergrid.

Photography Through the Operating Microscope. The operating laryngoscope that is used should have a nonreflecting matte inner surface. The monocular mirror-reflex camera is adapted to the beam splitter, the photoadapter, and the supplementary objective on the Zeiss operating microscope (Figure 9). The camera is provided with an automatic through-the-lens light meter, with a point or integrated light meter and a clear glass disc in the viewfinder. A winder and a cable release, or even better a foot switch, ensure that the photographs are free of blurring due to vibration. The larynx is illuminated solely by the halogen light of the operating microscope. Very careful adjustment and focusing of the operating microscope are essential to ensure that the image lies exactly in the middle of the frame. The focusing and magnification must be checked in the viewfinder of the reflex camera, because only that part of the image that appears in the eyepiece on the same side of the operating microscope is photographed. This part of the view does not coincide with the binocular image that the endoscopist sees. Focusing is carried out at high magnification with the help of a graticule.

During the exposure the patient's respiration must be arrested to prevent blurring due to movement. High-sensitivity artificial light film must be used to ensure that the exposure time is as brief as possible. The procedure is relatively simple and brief, and the views are highly magnified and fill the frame. The disadvantages include the patience and skill needed for focusing, uncontrollable chromatic aberration due

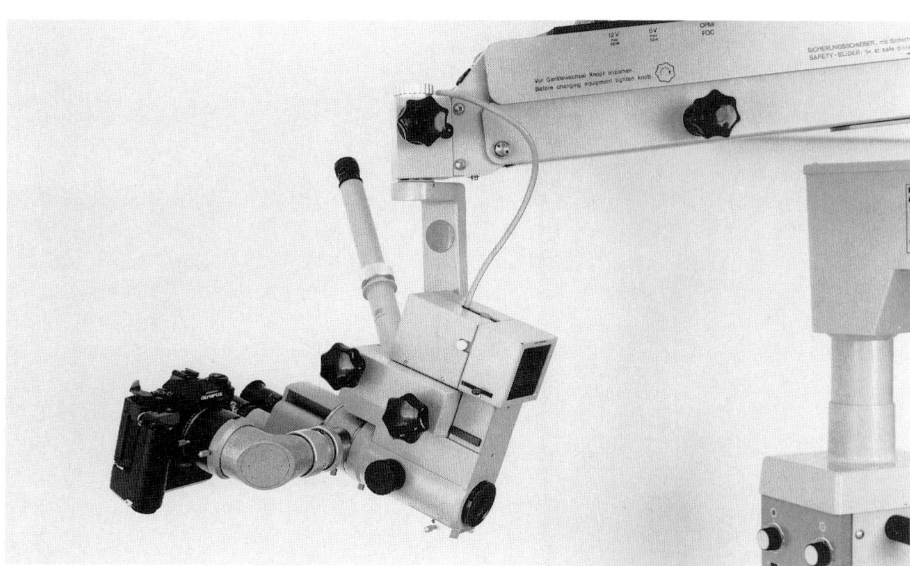

Fig. 9.

Laryngeal photography through the operating microscope. The automatically controlled through-the-lens camera is connected via a supplementary eyepiece to the photoadapter and the beam splitter. Illumination is provided by the halogen lamp in the operating microscope but may also be provided by distal illumination by a light carrier fixed to the laryngoscope. A computer flash is used as a light source.

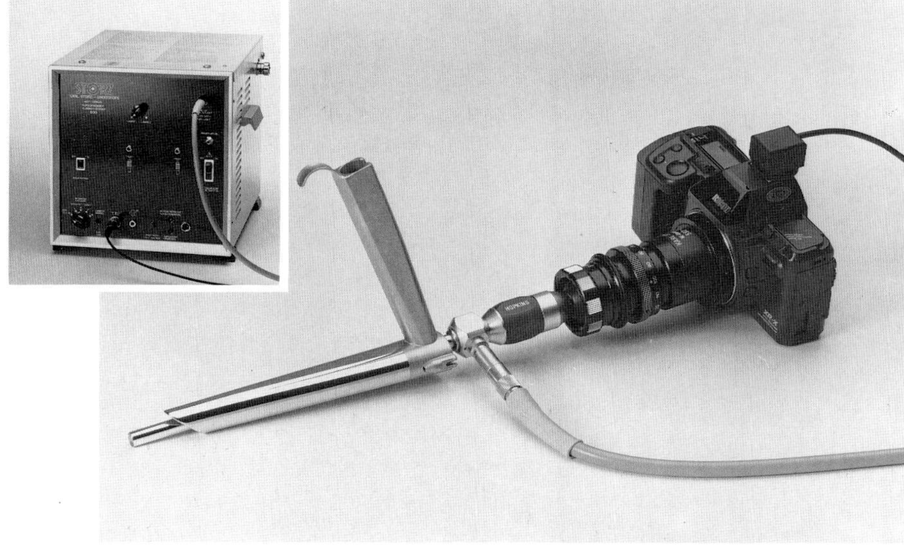

Fig. 10.

Laryngeal photography with a rod lens system. The wide-angled eyepiece of this apparatus with an integrated light carrier is introduced into the laryngoscope. The magnification of the view can be varied with a zoom lens. Illumination is provided by a computer flash source.

to varying potential and age of the lamp, and distortion of the quality of the view by reflections from the edge of the laryngoscope and from the cuff on the endotracheal tube. At higher magnifications the depth of focus is so small that it is often impossible to record the anterior and posterior parts of the vocal cord with equal sharpness. Fine blurring is frequent due to transmission of the patient's pulse beat to the larynx. However, most of the illustrations reproduced in this book have been taken by this method.

A computer flash as a light source combined with a through-the-lens reflex camera makes it possible to avoid movement-induced blurring of the photographs which are taken through the operating microscope. This method ensures optimal illumination of the object and avoidance of chromatic aberration due to varying tension of the lamp; moreover, a fine-grain daylight film may be used. Light is transported distally by a glass fiber to the point of the laryngoscope, or coaxially if the light carrier cable is incorporated in the lamp housing of the operating microscope by a special connector. This technique also has the disadvantage of difficult focusing and requires laborious checking of the view via the viewfinder of the camera.

Photography Using an Endoscopic Telescope Through the Operating Laryngoscope. In modern photographic endoscopes a wide-angled eyepiece that can be focused from several millimeters to infinity is integrated with a fiberglass carrier to a stable rod (Figure 10). This photographic laryngoscope is integrated with a monocular mirror-reflex camera that has a zoom objective and a through-the-lens light meter. The photographs are taken on daylight film, and lighting is provided by a computer-controlled flash. This photographic laryngoscope is the best current method of providing sharp pictures that are free of blurring and fill the slide. The magnification depends on the proximity of the objective to the subject and to what extent further magnification can be achieved with the proximal zoom objective. In addition to the 0° telescope of this photographic laryngoscope, angled 30° and 70° telescopes can be used for examining and photographing the anterior commissure and the lateral and infraglottic parts of the larynx (Figure 11).

Video Transmission and Recording. The large cameras used for the first teaching films of microlaryngoscopy have largely been replaced by modern videocameras. The small hand-held single-tube camera, or the newer, relatively insensitive, chip camera with a zoom objective, is fitted onto the small beam splitter and the video-adapter of the operating microscope (e.g., the Zeiss video-adapter F74 or F137). They can also be adapted directly or via a beam splitter to the laryngoscopic telescope or the fiberoptic laryngoscope (Figure 12). It is now almost always possible to show the patient his own larynx on the screen and to record this view by the use of modern videorecorders.

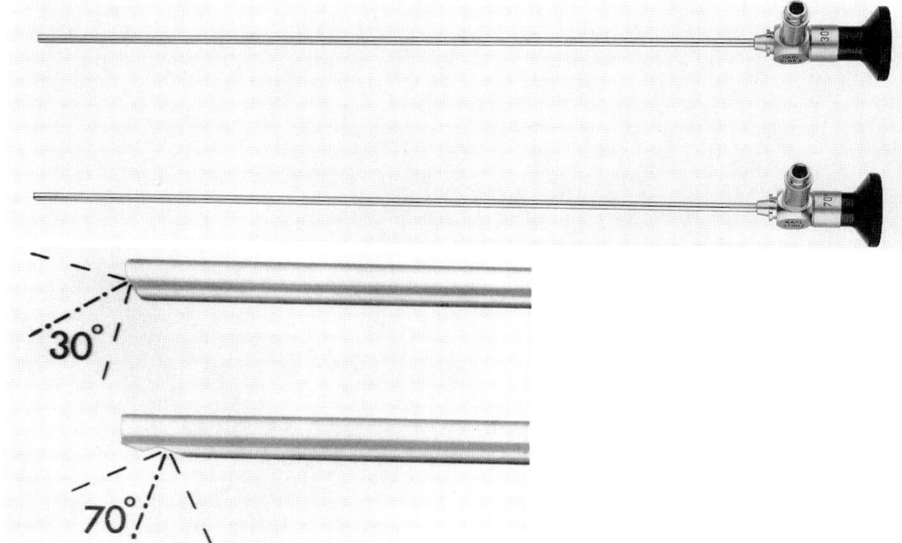

Fig. 11.

30° and 70° telescopes (Hopkins II) for inspection and photography of the lateral wall of the larynx, the ventricles and the subglottic space. These telescopes are introduced through the laryngoscope.

When making a videorecording through the operating microscope, it is irritating that only the part of the binocular field of vision seen in the ipsilateral eyepiece of the operating microscope appears on the screen. Thus, the view on the videoscreen does not correspond with the binocular view of the surgeon.

Berci and Kantor (personal communication, 1988) demonstrated an endoscopic telescope introduced laterally into the operating laryngoscope in a channel to which a videocamera can be connected. The surgeon can then carry out undisturbed binocular surgery using the operating microscope while the videocamera records the view from only a slightly different angle. It is even possible to abandon the operating microscope altogether and continue operating by monitoring the screen. The penalty of electronic image reproduction is a loss in detail reproduction, magnification, and color fidelity. The quality of the image produced by modern videocameras is outstanding but is not as good as that achieved through an endoscopic telescope or an operating microscope. However, the purpose of a video-camera is to of an operation and not to produce a sharp still picture that is accurate to the last detail.

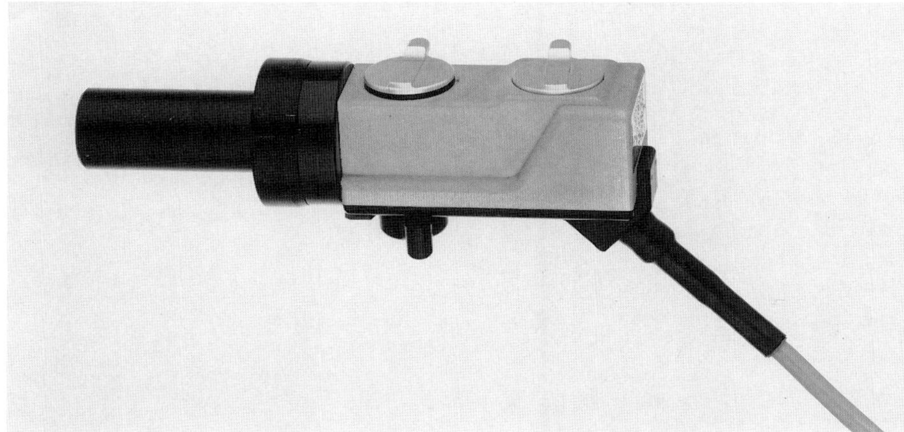

Fig. 12.

Chip video camera (Storz Endovision 534) with monitor and recorder for adaptation to the operating microscope, the telescope, the fiberoptic laryngoscope, the endoscopic eye piece, or the observation arm.

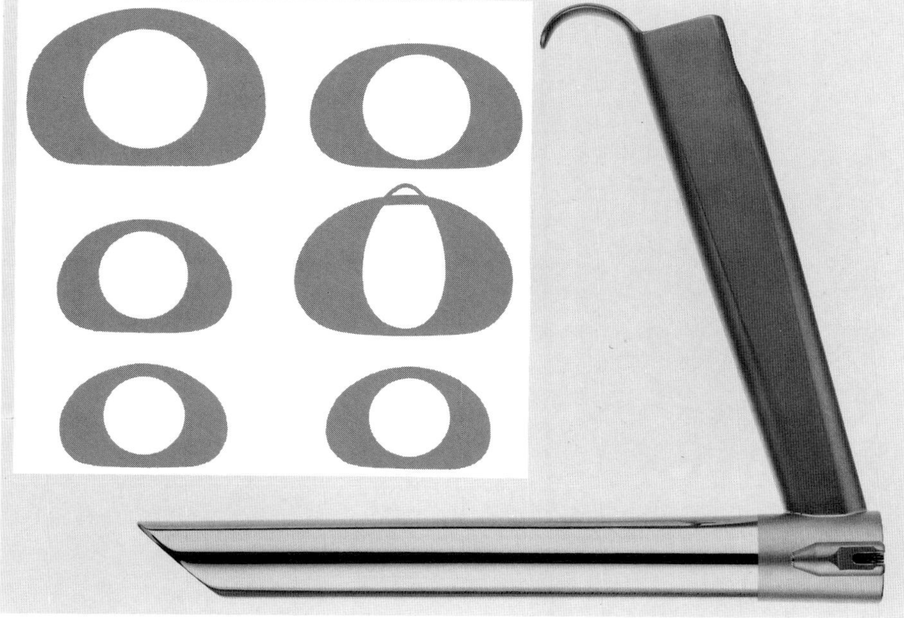

Fig. 13.

Laryngoscopes of varying sizes and lengths for adults and children. The diameter of the proximal opening is shown in its natural size. All operating laryngoscopes have a flat surface to distribute pressure evenly over the teeth.

3. Instruments for Microlaryngoscopy and Endolaryngeal Microsurgery

As the surgeon's experience increases, he needs fewer and fewer instruments, even for the most difficult procedures, and should confine himself to a few simple, robust instruments that are easy to sterilize. The number of instruments in the set that I developed with Storz has decreased during the last 30 years; oldfashioned instruments have been improved and only a few new instruments have been added.

A set of operating laryngoscopes of varying sizes suffices for all conditions (Figure 13). I generally use laryngoscopes C and B for adults, and these are suitable for about 80% of all examinations. The narrow DN model is suitable for restricted access and can be used through a gap in the teeth. If the patient's neck is unusually long, it may be necessary to use a long laryngoscope. If the anterior commissure is difficult to expose or can only be brought into view with excessive pressure, an instrument such as Holinger's anterior commissure laryngoscope, whose point curves upwards anteriorly, may be useful. A set of smaller children's laryngoscopes is also available, together with a correspondingly short chest support and instruments, but the adult instruments can be used on most patients above the age of 7.

All my operating laryngoscopes have a broad, flat surface to distribute the pressure over the teeth of the upper jaw so that it is not concentrated on one point of the teeth or the gums. The internal surface of the laryngoscopes is matted to prevent the reflexion of light.

Other laryngoscopes commercially available include those with a highly curved point, those with oval or round openings, and the split distending laryngoscope, but I have no personal experience with these instruments.

Distal illumination is usually provided by fiberoptic light carriers (Figure 14). Proximal illumination can be achieved by an attached prism. I usually use a light carrier to introduce the laryngoscope and then immediately remove it after exposure of the larynx. Excellent illumination is thereafter provided exclusively by the operating microscope, even when access is restricted and when working at great depth.

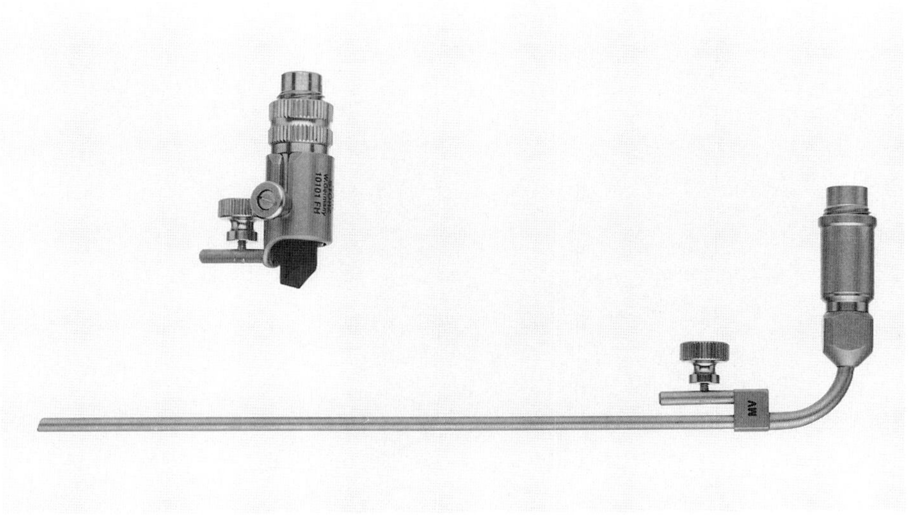

Fig. 14.

Light carrier for distal and proximal illumination for adaptation to the operating microscope. Light is reflected through a prism when using proximal illumination. The light carrier is usually removed after introduction and fixation of the laryngoscope, because the light from the microscope suffices for examination and surgery.

The breast support has undergone almost no change for several decades (Figure 15). The support consists either of a wide-diameter rubber ring or two pads. Placing the breast support on a separate table is a cumbersome and superfluous procedure, at least for adults; several thousand microlaryngoscopies have shown that the patient's respiration is in practice very little influenced by placing the support immediately on the chest. A further advantage is that the support can be moved on the thorax while the head is moved in the opposite direction to achieve a better view of the lateral walls of the larynx. I now use a separate table for the chest support in infants and young children only.

The teeth or the edentulous alveolus should always be protected against the pressure of the laryngoscope, preferably by using a dental impression plate, which is available in several sizes (Figure 16a). The impression plate distributes the pressure evenly over the teeth and gums, bridges any gaps between the teeth, and prevents cracking of the enamel. Gum shields consisting of soft plastic or rubber do indeed protect the enamel but do not distribute the pressure of the laryngoscope, and are not to be recommended.

I use exclusively the universal Zeiss operating microscope with a hand-driven zoom fitted with a 400 mm or a 375 mm objective. A long focal length is necessary to provide a sufficiently long working distance for manipulation of the long-handled instruments.

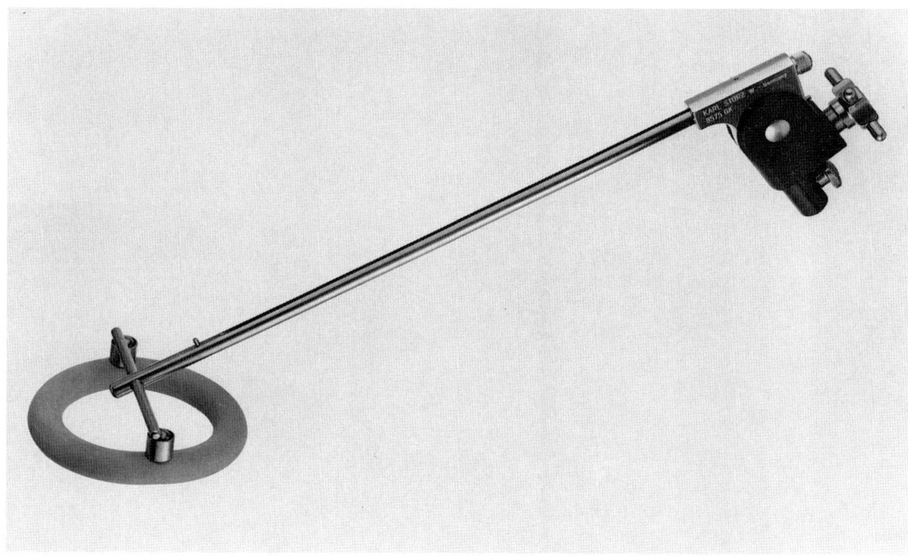

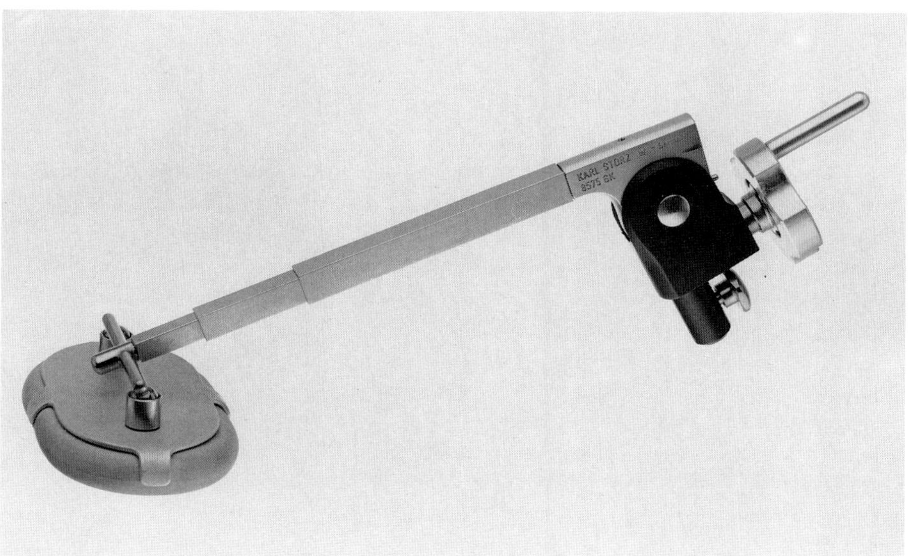

Fig. 15.

Breastplate (chest holder) for children and adults.

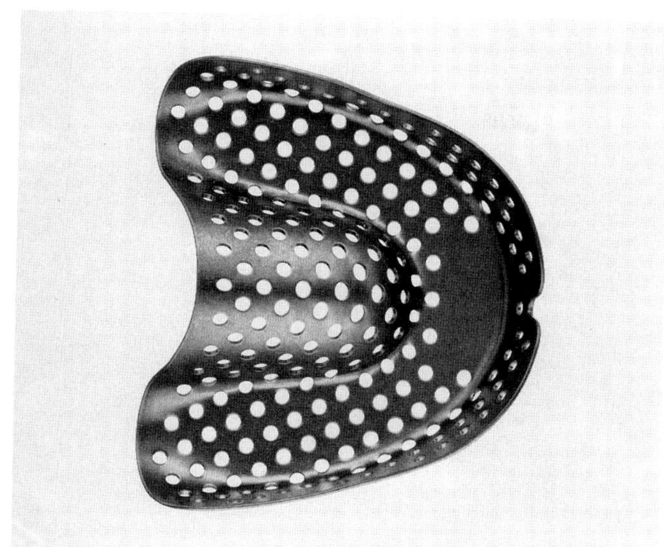

Fig. 16 a.

Dental impression plate distributing the pressure of the laryngoscope evenly on the upper teeth and hard palate. The impression plate bridges any gaps in the teeth.

Fig. 16 b, c, d.

Cupped forceps (16b), alligator forceps (16c) and scissors (16d) with various directions of jaws and in different sizes and lengths for children and adults.

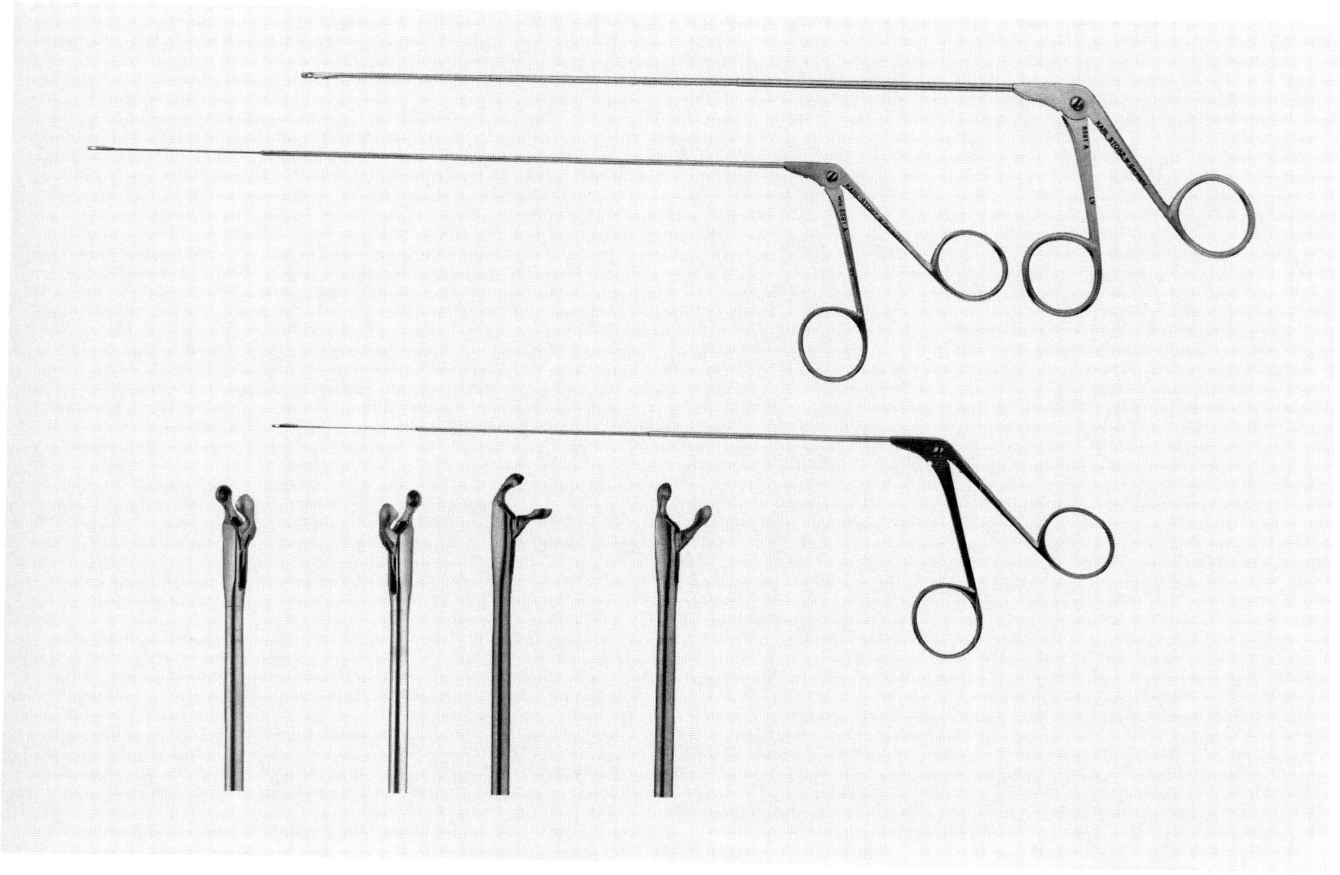

Small forceps and scissors (Figure 16d) with jaws of varying size and a working distance of about 22 cm (less in children) are the main instruments to be used. The instruments are available in three sizes, but the largest cupped forceps are only used occasionally for biopsy of large tumors (Figure 16b). The cupped forceps and the fine alligator forceps are mainly used for grasping and holding, and not for the nipping off or tearing off of tissue! Small forceps and scissors may be straight, curved upwards, or curved concavely to the right or left.

I seldom use a knife, and then only a slightly curved knife fitted to an interchangeable handgrip (Figure 17). Suction tubes of varying diameters are isolated as far as the tip so that they can be used simultaneously with diathermy to suck off the smoke (Figure 17).

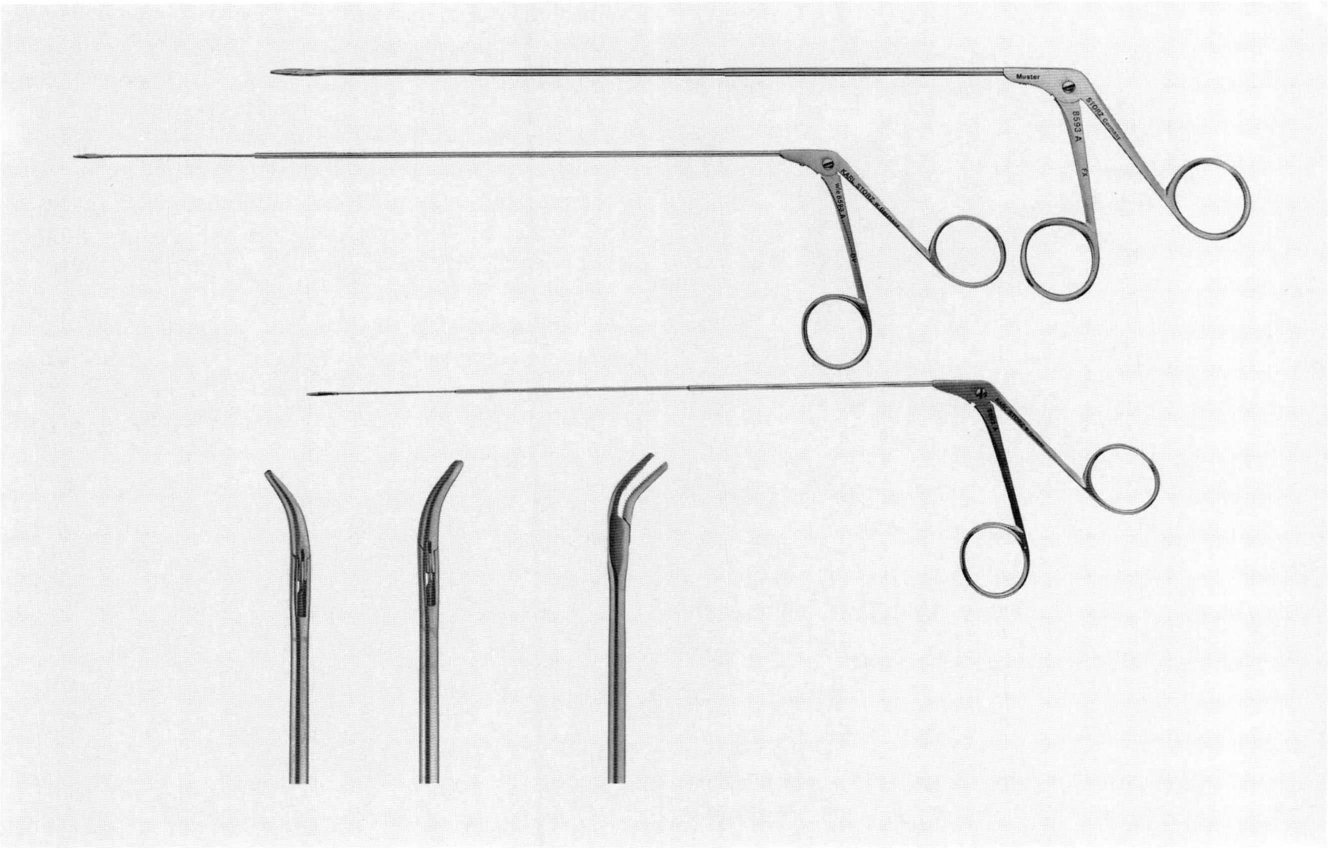

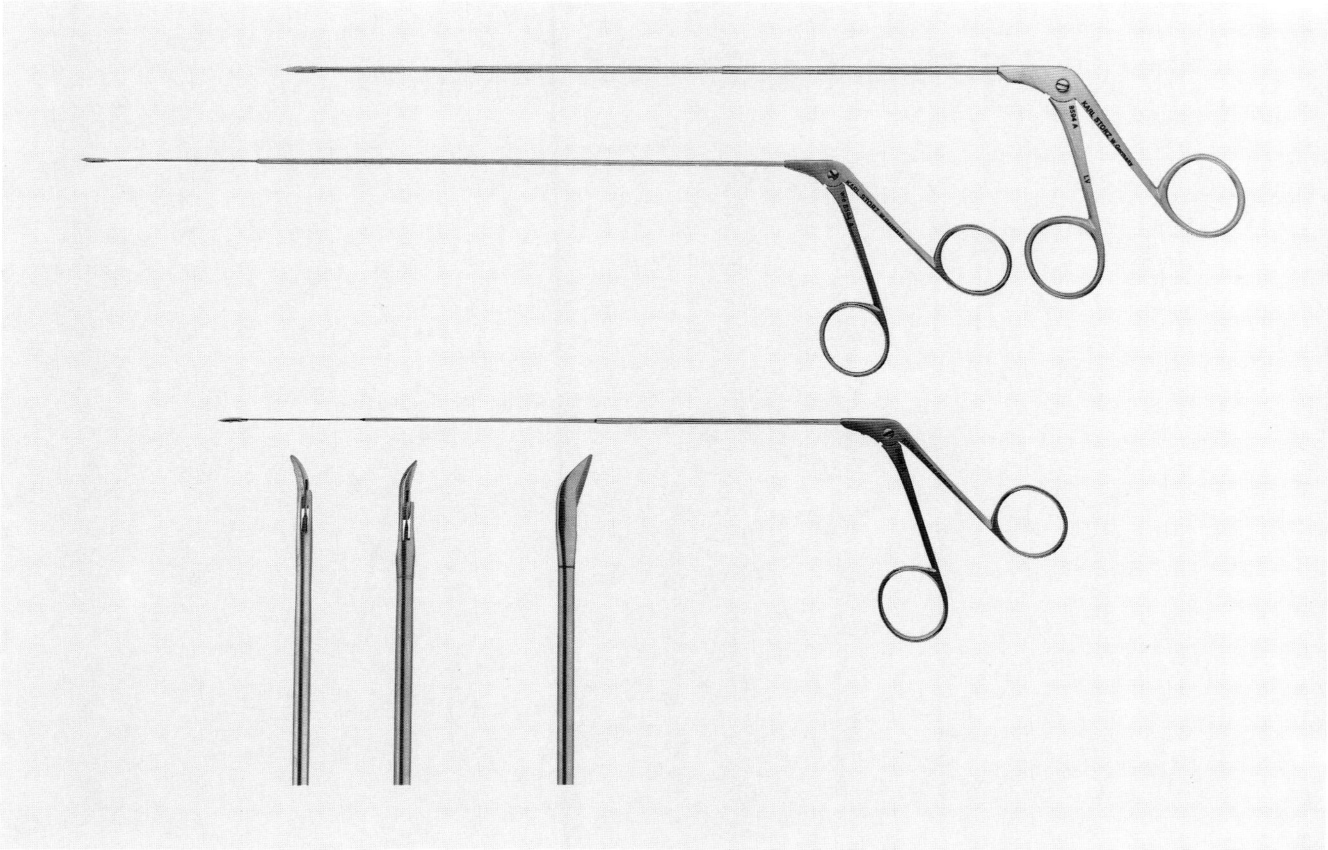

Electrocoagulation for hemostasis or suction coagulation and diathermy dissection are carried out with microcoagulators and fine needles of various sizes.

The microcoagulators and dissectors are connected to a high-frequency, processor-controlled electrosurgical unit (Figure 18). After application of an alternating current of more than 300,000 Hz, the ions of the tissue fluid begin to resonate at the frequency of the electric current. This produces a thermal effect that evaporates the water of the intra- and extracellular fluids under a relatively slow heating of the tissue, producing contraction of the coagulable tissues such as the vessel walls. This contraction effect is used for hemostasis. If the tissue is heated more rapidly, the temperature of the cell fluids rises so quickly that the pressure of the steam ruptures the cell walls and the tissue splits. The high-frequency electrosurgical unit so far has the disadvantage of uncontrolled formation of electric sparks and arcs. A newer model corrects the high frequency cutting current after measurement of tissue resistance. It does this so quickly that the same reproducible quality of incision is always achieved, despite a varying depth of cut and varying flexibility and conductivity of the tissue. The pulsed current turns itself off automatically before the tissue undergoes carbonization.

The high-frequency, processor-controlled electrosurgical unit has the advantages that its price is relatively moderate, that it requires no additional safety measures for the prevention of reflexion and burns (as is the case with laser devices), and that it can also be used for coagulation in relatively inaccessible angles and niches.

The use of a laser in endolaryngeal microsurgery has been recommended enthusiastically.[19] I feel that the decision as to whether to use a laser or not should be left to the individual, once he is able to use the instrument accurately and carefully.[25] Having watched several prominent users of the laser at work, I am convinced that practically all endolaryngeal microsurgical procedures can be carried out more quickly, more accurately, and less traumatically without the laser. It is certainly wrong to believe that operations which are difficult with conventional instruments can be carried out more easily with the laser. I regard vaporization of benign lesions causing dysphonia, such as nodules, polyps, and cysts, as incorrect, because there is then no opportunity to submit tissue for histologic examination.

Fig. 17.

Knives of various types on an interchangeable handgrip. The suction tubes, of various sizes, must be isolated as far as the tip so that they can be used simultaneously with electrocoagulation.

All instruments that generate heat – be it high-frequency coagulators or laser beams – produce a burn that heals less well than a smooth incision. An increasing number of voices have been raised, not least by voice therapists, warning against the use of the laser. It has not been shown that the laser achieves better results in the removal of papillomas, nor is its use attended by fewer recurrences than the use of the high-frequency suction coagulation apparatus. A laser is not absolutely necessary for resection of a vocal cord, and furthermore a deep resection into the vocal cord musculature should not be carried out by endolaryngeal microsurgery.

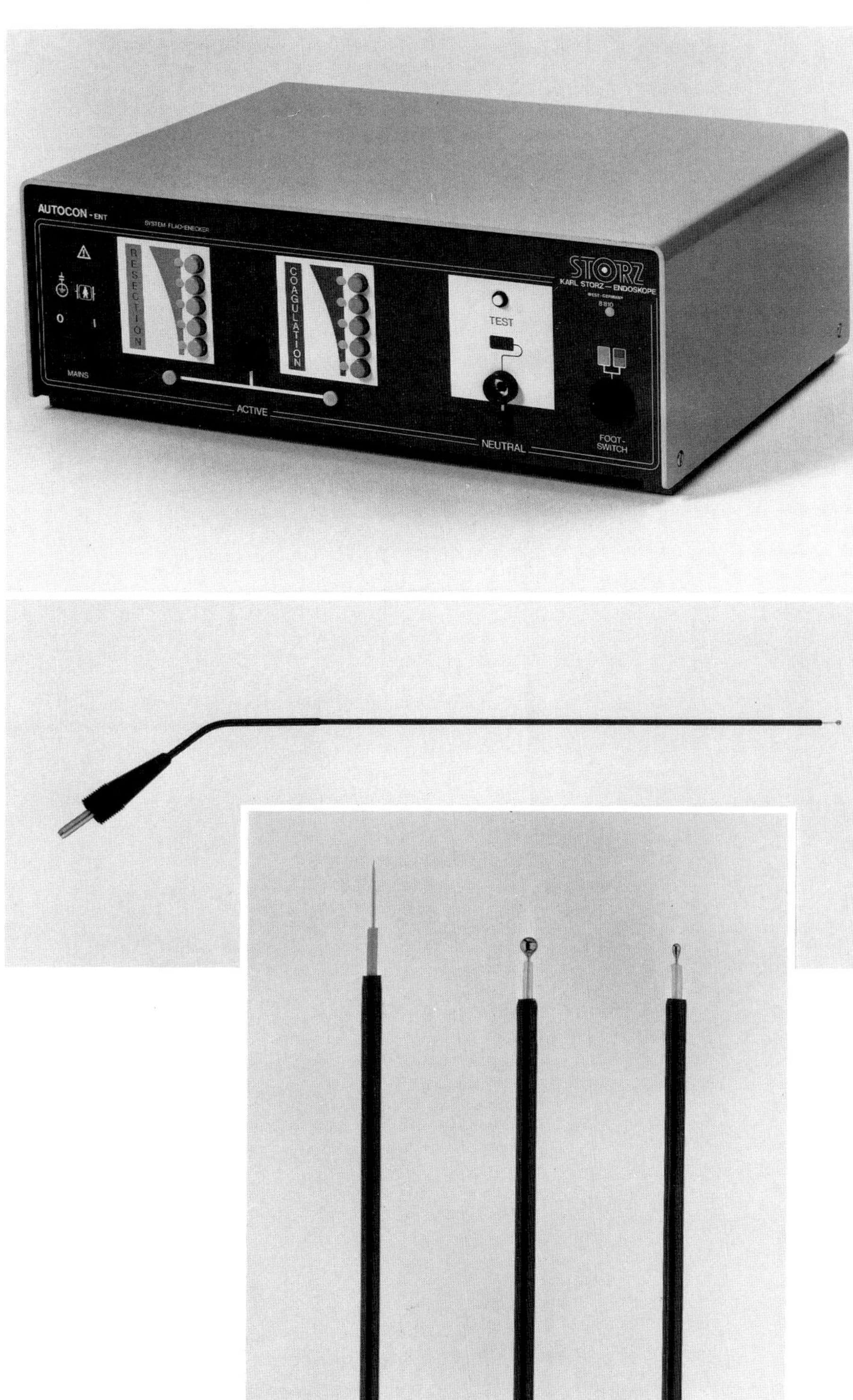

Fig. 18.

Microcoagulator and needle microdissector for hemostasis and electrosurgery. A processor-controlled, high-frequency electrosurgical unit is used as the energy source.

4. Indications, Contraindications, and Preoperative Procedures

Microlaryngoscopy and endolaryngeal microsurgery demand general anesthesia and can therefore lead to serious complica- desirable to weigh carefully the pros and cons of such an operation, and to record in detail the preoperative findings and any discussion with the patient.

Many patients ask **when** the examination and the operation have to be carried out. If a premalignant or malignant lesion is suspected, the examination is urgently required, of course. But even benign lesions should be operated on as soon as possible because patients with polyps or cysts of a vocal cord often develop contact reactions, such as pits, edema, and epithelial thickening, on the contralateral cord, and these are sometimes not controllable by surgery. Even stenotic lesions may require an early operation.

In many years of experience I have never seen resolution of an organic lesion such as a polyp, a cyst, a vocal cord nodule, or a varix achieved by voice therapy, electrical treatment, or other nonsurgical means. Also, voice exercises do not achieve any improvement in bilateral vocal cord paresis. Such useless and superfluous voice exercises only prolong the disability and treatment unnecessarily, and hinder restoration of the voice. **The proper time for voice therapy is the postoperative period.**

In some patients, acute inflammatory laryngeal lesions demand initial conservative treatment, for example with inhalation therapy.

Microlaryngoscopy is contraindicated if general anesthesia is a threat to the patient's life, for example after a recent infarct, in patients with aneurysms, bradycardia, etc. Of course an increased risk is justified in patients with suspected malignancy, but in low-risk cases microlaryngoscopy should be omitted in favor of an indirect biopsy or biopsy via a fiberoptic laryngoscope.

Microlaryngoscopy may be technically impossible if the cervical spine cannot be extended, as in ankylosing spondylitis or fracture of the cervical spine, in mandibular deformities, and in patients with a short thick neck associated with marked prognathism. However, an experienced surgeon encounters such cases relatively seldom. Most cases that have been referred to me because microlaryngoscopy could not be carried out elsewhere proved to be suitable for microlaryngoscopy without particular difficulty provided the technical rules of the modality were observed.

The possibility of local complications must be dealt with during the preoperative discussion (page 29), and patients with stenosis, trauma, or tumor narrowing the larynx must be warned of the possibility of prolonged intubation or tracheotomy.

Almost all patients are anxious to know the postoperative quality of their voice. They should be told that restitution of their normal voice may require several weeks, and that voice therapy may sometimes be necessary to achieve normalization. The voice may be higher or lower after the operation, or it may show other changes. In some patients undergoing removal of multiple papillomas or extensive vocal cord excision for small carcinomas or chronic laryngitis, it is predictable that their postoperative voice will be satisfactory for everyday purposes, but that they will no longer have a normal voice, especially not a singing voice. A careful discussion of the prospects for voice improvement is necessary with patients who use their voice professionally, e.g., teachers and business people. Singers and actors need an especially frank and detailed counseling because their careers depend on a normal voice.

Nowadays it is easy to compare the voice before and after operation by means of standard texts and with simple melodies using a tape recorder. However, this comparison of an often abnormal voice both before and after operation is largely a subjective decision. Many voices are no longer comparable, for example, before and after removal of Reinke's edema. Sadly, there is still no straightforward standardized procedure for measuring vocal function and for recording it simply (similar to an audiogram) to allow comparison with an ideal normal voice.[17]

5. Anesthesia

Close cooperation between the laryngologist and the anesthesiologist is a prerequisite for successful endolaryngeal microsurgery. The anesthesia must be as safe and pleasant as possible for the patient, must be simple to monitor by the anesthesiologist, and must allow the surgeon to work unhindered and unhurried on a completely relaxed patient. These conditions are best achieved by endotracheal anesthesia through a thin endotracheal catheter, along with a relaxant and positive pressure respiration.

Every anesthesiologist has his own preferred premedication, but this should always include atropine. During intubation and also during introduction of the laryngoscope the blood pressure rises and the pulse quickens, but in many patients the blood pressure may fall and the pulse slow, or arrythmias may arise, probably elicited by the laryngeal reflex. Therefore, it is advisable to spray the hypopharynx and the larynx with a topical anesthetic such as lidocaine to eliminate this reflex.

Anesthesia is induced by intravenous injection of a barbiturate or by application of a gas mixture via a mask. Relaxation is usually achieved by a bolus of succinylcholine. The surgeon can recognize when the relaxant is wearing off by the return of spontaneous movements of the vocal cord or by swallowing movements, and he should warn the anesthesiologist of this. A long-term relaxant is to be preferred for prolonged operations, such as arytenoidectomy or cordectomy.

A cuffed Woodbridge catheter is used for the intubation: a size Charrier 28 is usually used for men and a Ch 24–26 for women. Catheters of size Ch 18–20 may be used for children and patients with small or narrow larynges. Pollard's catheter is particularly useful; it is thinned over only a short segment distally, thus leaving more room in the larynx for manipulation, but interfering only slightly with the respiratory resistance (Figure 19).[23]

The anesthetic usually consists of a gas mixture such as halothane, nitrous oxide, and oxygen. Respiration is usually carried out mechanically with positive pressure.

The anesthesia should be deep but is usually not required for a long time, the average operating time being about 15 minutes and in many cases 6 to 7 minutes. Operations lasting one hour are very unusual.

Alternatives to intubation anesthesia have been proposed, such as apneic oxygenation, topical anesthesia, and blockade of the superior laryngeal nerve. Jet ventilation using a thin jet lying in front of or within the larynx demands a particularly well-trained anesthesiologist and good collaboration with the surgeon.

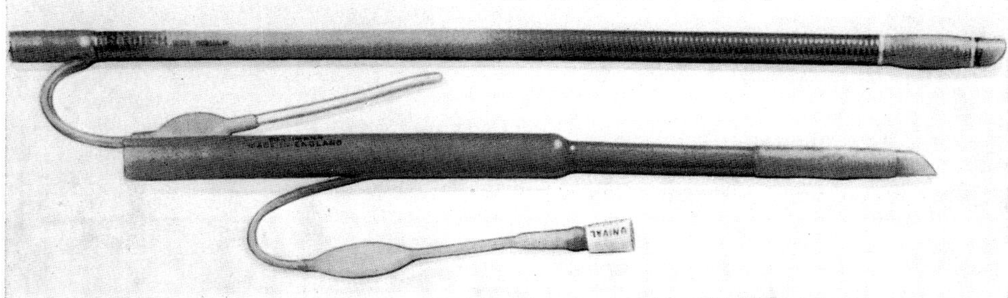

Fig. 19.

Woodbridge and Pollard endotracheal tubes in sizes between Charrier 20 and 28 guarantee satisfactory ventilation and also leave sufficient space within the larynx for the surgeon.

6. Technique of Microlaryngoscopy

The training of many colleagues in the technique of microlaryngoscopy has shown that this technique is more difficult to learn than might be thought and therefore demands thorough description.

The correct position of the patient is a prerequisite for optimal introduction of the laryngoscope. It is possible in many cases to carry out microlaryngoscopy with the head elevated or extended, but such a procedure often does not provide a satisfactory view of the larynx. The patient should preferably lie flat on a horizontal operating table, with neither head rings nor sand bags under the shoulders (Figure 20).

The dental plate is put in place before the laryngoscope is introduced (Figure 21). If individual teeth are particularly at risk, the dental plate can be supplemented with impression material to protect these teeth more effectively. The edentulous jaw is protected with a rubber plate if greater than normal pressure will be needed on the laryngoscope.

The laryngoscope is only introduced when the patient is fully relaxed and sufficiently anesthetized.

The largest possible laryngoscope is chosen that will give a good view of the larynx, reflect as much light as possible into the larynx, and will allow the best photographs to be taken. The surgeon very rapidly learns how to estimate which laryngoscope is the most suitable for individual anatomical conditions and should not hesitate to use a smaller instrument or a special scope if a wide-caliber endoscope requires the use of force for its introduction.

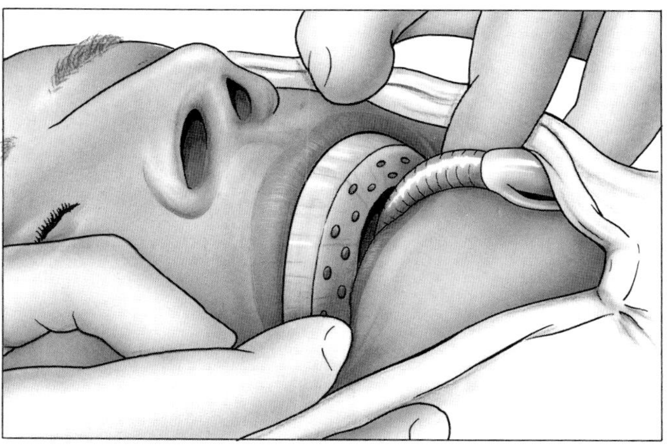

Fig. 21.

Insertion of the protective dental plate.

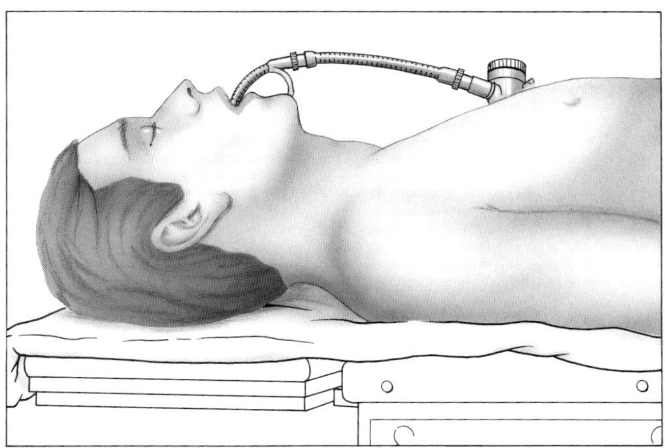

Fig. 20.

Correct positioning at the start of the procedure with the patient lying flat on a horizontal operating table. Note that no head ring is used, and the head is neither elevated nor hanging.

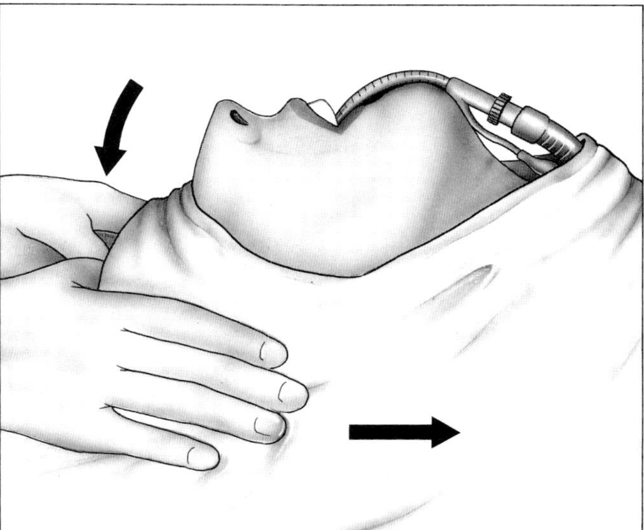

Fig. 22.

Maximal retroflexion of the patient's head under relaxation before insertion of the laryngoscope.

Before introducing the laryngoscope, the patient's head is fully extended (Figure 22). A laryngoscope is now introduced between the endotracheal tube behind and the lower jaw in front, taking care not to crush the lip or the tongue against the dental plate or the teeth (Figure 23). After the mucus has been sucked out of the pharynx, the laryngoscope is pushed forward, following the endotracheal tube between the epiglottis and the tube, until its point reaches the petiole of the epiglottis. The laryngoscope should be pushed forward with a smooth movement and not with a levering action. If the laryngoscope is passed too deeply into the larynx, both the vestibular folds and the vocal cords are displaced laterally, whereas if the scope is not passed deeply enough the vestibular folds obscure the vocal cords (Figure 24). Once the laryngoscope is in the correct position, the chest holder is put in place, the supporting rod extended, and the laryngoscope fixed in its position by a few turns on the adjusting screw (Figure 25). After exact adjustment of the scope, both vocal cords can now be seen as far as the apex of the vocal process. The endotracheal tube is pushed into the posterior commissure, and thus out of the operating field, by the back wall of the laryngoscope. At the same time the vocal cords are put under slight tension, facilitating surgical manipulations (Figure 26).

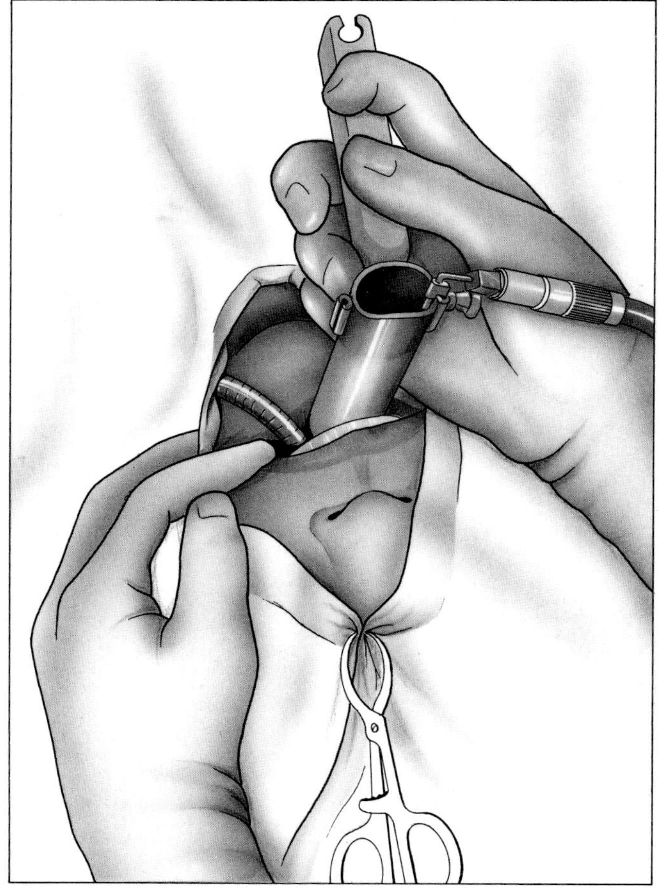

Fig. 23.

Introduction of the operating laryngoscope, taking care not to catch the lips or the tongue between the teeth. The laryngoscope should be introduced smoothly and not be pushed forward by levering movements.

If the posterior part of the larynx requires attention, for example for the removal of a contact granuloma, the endotracheal tube is pushed into the anterior commissure with the tip of the laryngoscope (Figure 27).

External pressure on the larynx by an assistant helps to avoid the use of excessive pressure on the laryngoscope (Figure 28). The entire larynx can be pushed posteriorly or displaced to one or the other side to obtain a better view of the anterior commissure or the lateral wall of the larynx. The surgeon can correct the pressure exerted by the assistant's hand to ensure that the larynx is brought fully into view.

A better view of the anterior commissure can often be obtained by retracting the point of the laryngoscope to the level of the vestibular folds and then increasing the external pressure on the inferior part of the larynx to bring the larynx into an obtuse angle with the optical axis of the laryngoscope, which improves the field of vision. In addition to the use of special laryngoscopes such as the DN and anterior commissure scopes, there is another solution for the larynx that is difficult to expose: the laryngoscope is introduced obliquely through the angle of the mouth with the extended head turned slightly to one side, and then it is introduced into the larynx between the tongue and tonsil (Figure 29). In this position, however, the pressure of the laryngoscope often tears the palate and the lateral pharyngeal wall.

Experience and practice are needed to expose the larynx in difficult anatomical conditions, but ultimately it is very unusual not to obtain a satisfactory view. Once the laryngoscope is fixed in the desired position, the light carrier is removed and the operating microscope brought in. Illumination is now provided exclusively by the light from the operating microscope. Focusing now follows under high magnification.

The 30° or 70° angled telescope introduced through the laryngoscope can be used with advantage to examine the laryngeal surface of the epiglottis, the lateral wall of the larynx, or the subglottic space (page 9).

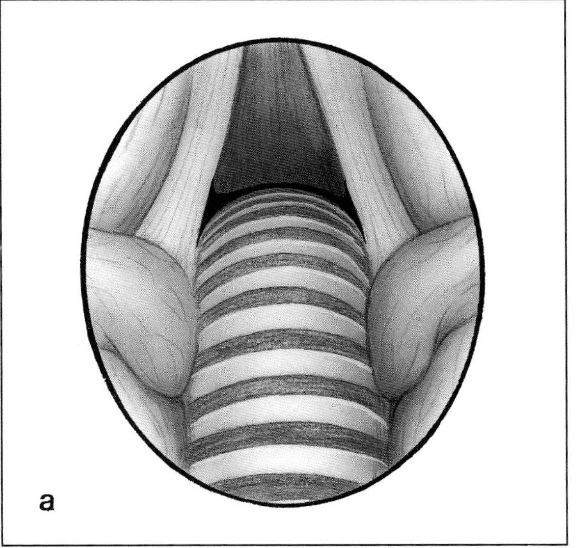

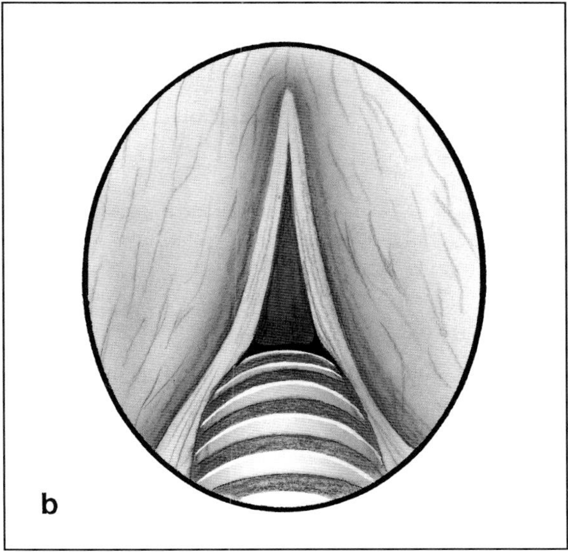

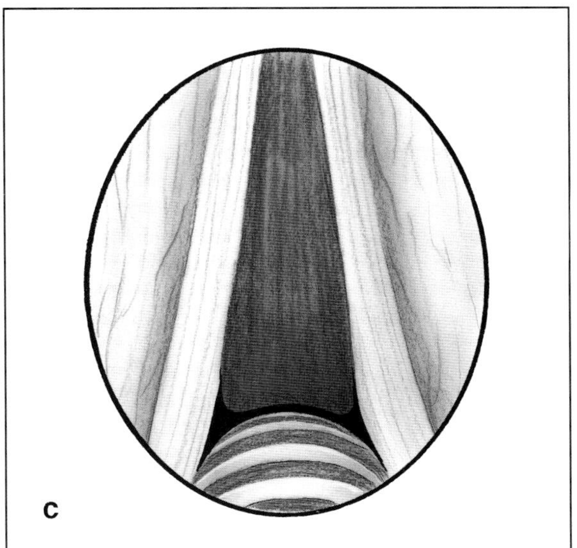

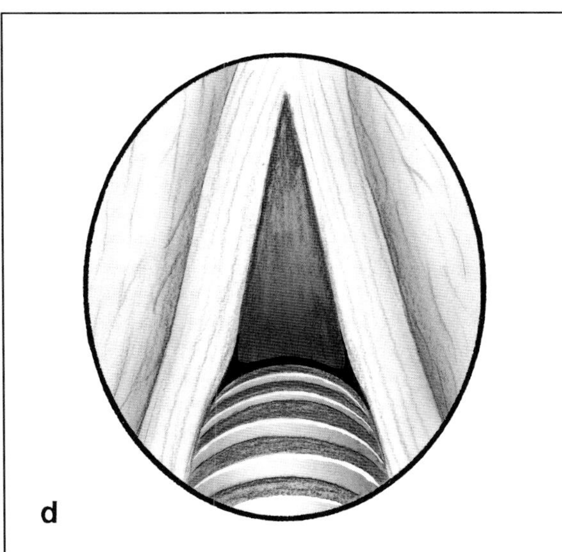

Fig. 24.

Visible part of the larynx with varying adjustment of the laryngoscope:
a. The tip of the laryngoscope has not yet been introduced far enough to demonstrate the anterior part of the vocal cords.
b. The laryngoscope has not been introduced deeply enough into the larynx; the vestibular folds are still obscuring the vocal cords
c. The laryngoscope has been introduced too far into the larynx and its tip pushes the vocal cords to the side.
d. Optimal adjustment of the laryngoscope for examination of the vocal cords.

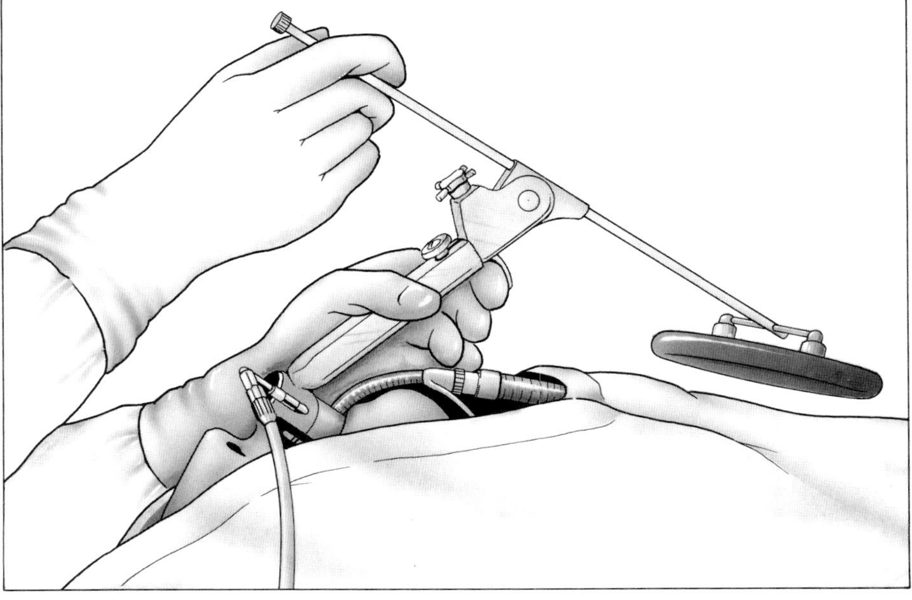

Fig. 25.

Once the laryngoscope is in the correct position, the chest holder is applied and the rod extended.

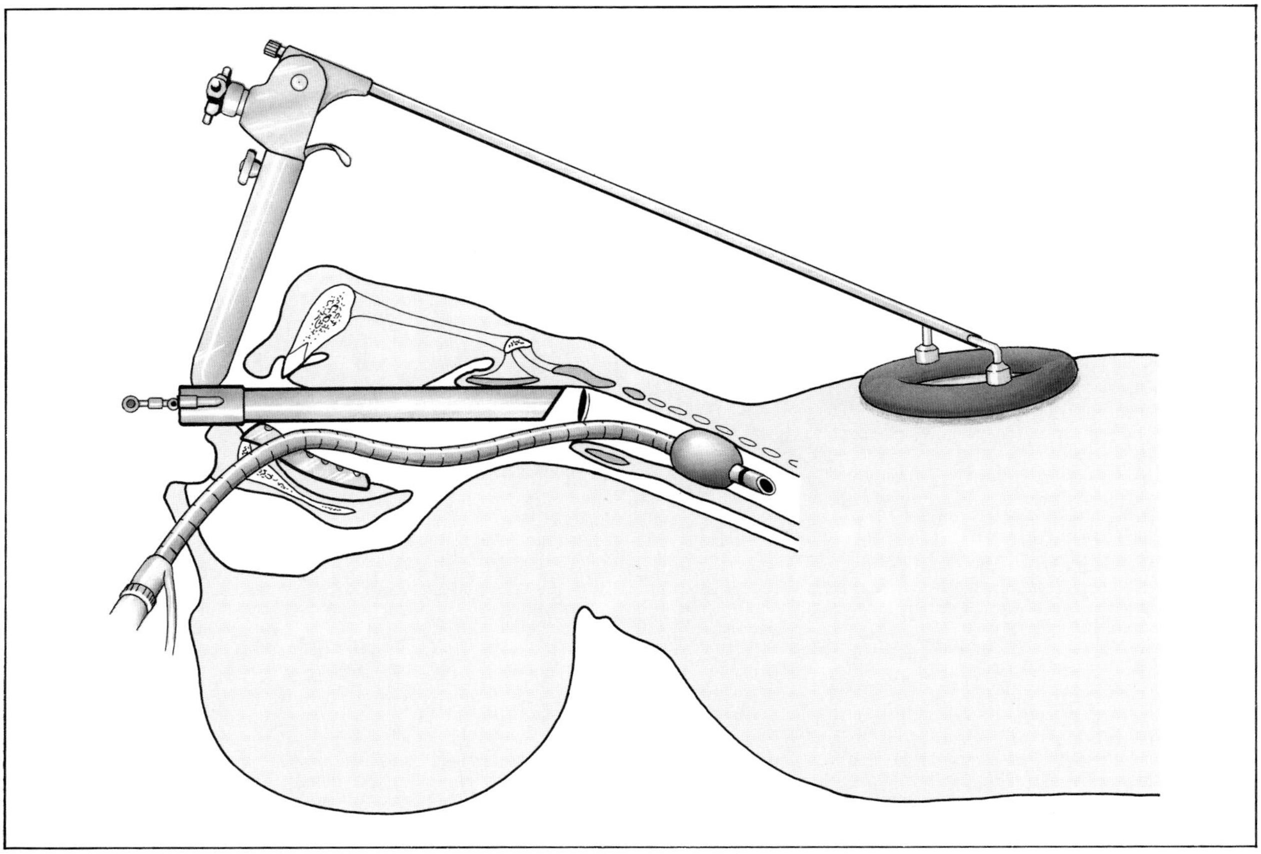

Fig. 26.

Correct adjustment of the laryngoscope for the first phase of microlaryngoscopy.

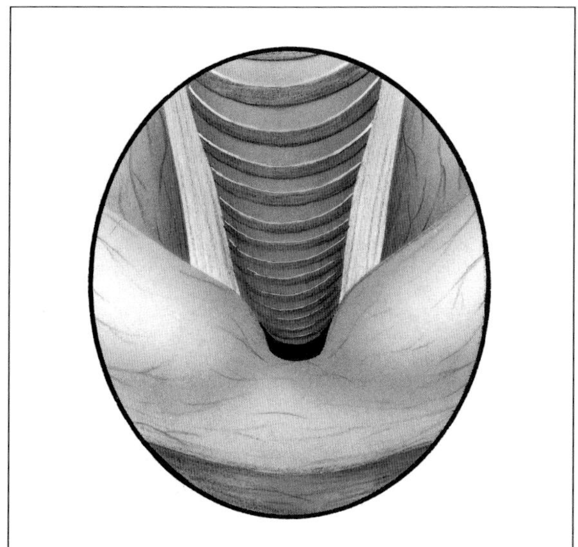

Fig. 27.

Position of the laryngoscope for an operation in the posterior segment of the larynx: the endotracheal tube has been pushed into the anterior commissure with the tip of the laryngoscope.

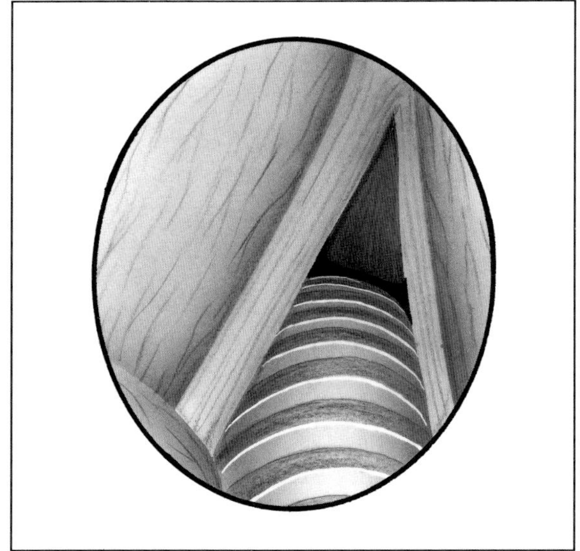

Fig. 28.

An assistant pushes the larynx backwards or to the side with his hand for better demonstration of individual parts of the larynx without increasing the pressure of the laryngoscope.

During the examination, the surgeon should be sitting upright and relaxed. Sitting bent forward or over-extended because the operating table or the surgeon's stool is too high or too low produces unnecessary tension and cramp (Figure 30).

Once the examination is finished the larynx and hypopharynx are carefully sucked clear of mucus and blood. The adjusting screw of the chest holder is loosened, the rods are withdrawn, and the laryngoscope is removed. The pharynx and the teeth should be checked carefully for damage before the patient recovers from the anesthesia.

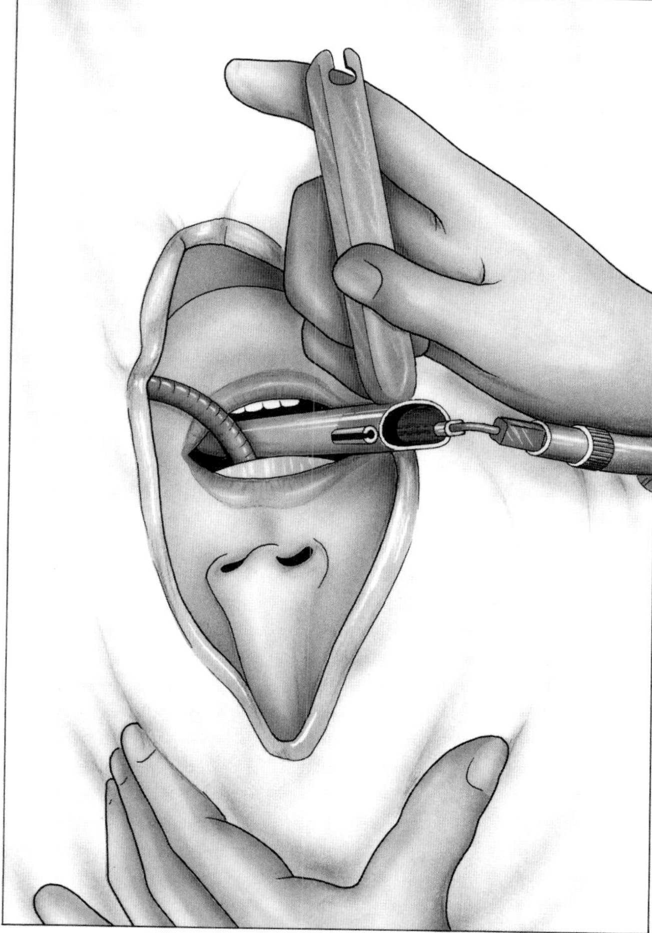

Fig. 29.

Introduction of the laryngoscope via the angle of the mouth on the right side with the head turned slightly to the left. This position can be used for larynges that are difficult to expose but provides a good view of only one-half of the larynx.

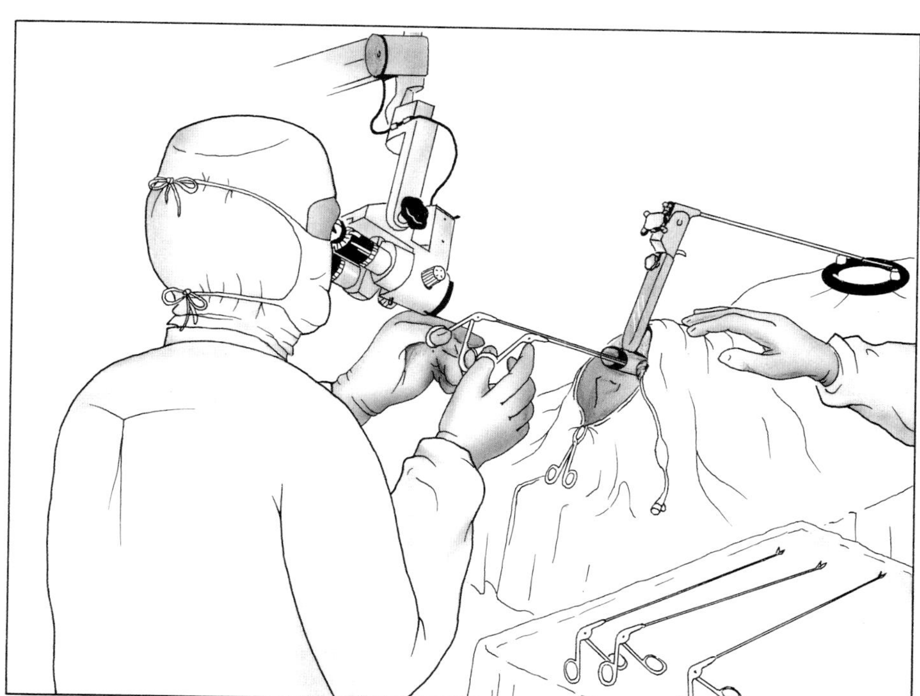

Fig. 30.

An endolaryngeal microsurgical procedure. The surgeon should sit upright with his body relaxed and allow his elbows to hang down.

7. Technique of Endolaryngeal Operations

The function of the larynx as the transmitter of speech and diverse emotional utterances demands the same respect as as does the function of the eye and the ear, the other organs of communication. The vocal cords are sensitive organs, and surgery should be as conservative and as precise as that of the mucosa of the middle ear. Sadly, many patients are seen with defects, irregular surfaces, scars, and adhesions of the vocal cord which cause irreparable postoperative dysphonia. It is true that such operative sequelae cannot always be avoided if the type and extent of the disease necessitate an extensive procedure, but these sequelae can be minimized by experience and exact surgical technique.

The beginner is strongly advised to practice the use of the long-handled fine instruments first on a model. My own trainees practice on a laryngoscope mounted in a support, using the operating microscope with a 400 mm objective. A cadaver larynx, a glove finger filled with gauze, or a similar object is fastened in front of the tip of the laryngoscope to allow all minor operations to be simulated.

It is an important basic principle that surgery should always be carried out with both hands using two instruments (Figure 31).

Dissection is usually carried out using a combination of a small forceps and scissors, or a suction tube and a coagulator. Small forceps are used for grasping material such as a polyp but not for plucking off, tearing, nipping off, or stripping tissue. It is a basic error of technique to nip or tear off a polyp, nodule, cyst, or Reinke's edema, since this leaves jagged mucosal edges causing irregular surfaces on the vocal cord.[38] Dissection may be carried too deeply in this type of surgery, tearing or even removing fibers of the vocal ligament; it is virtually impossible later to fill out a defect, particularly on the vocal cords.

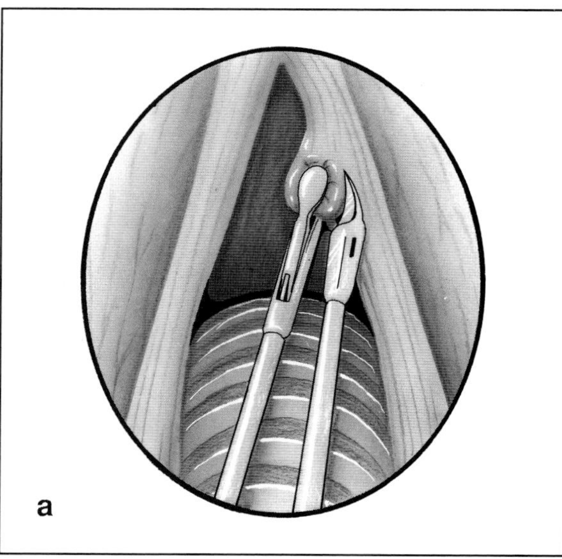

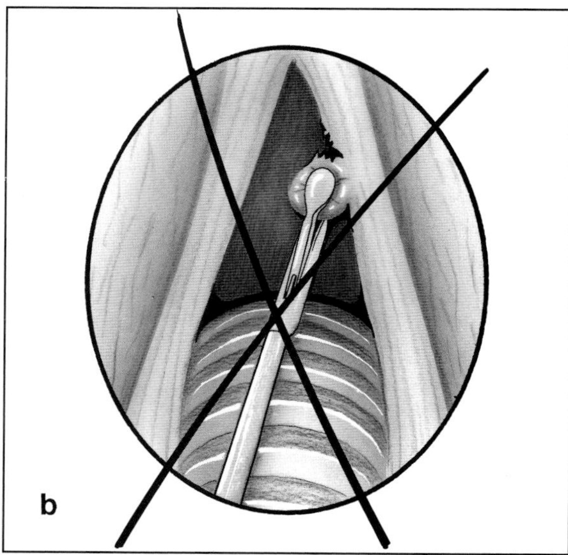

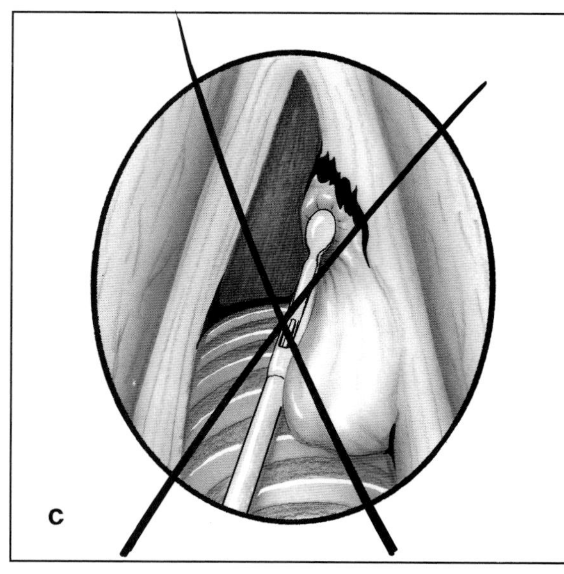

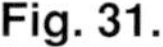

Fig. 31.

As a matter of principle, two instruments should always be used for surgery:
a. One instrument is used to grasp the object, and the second is used for dissection or cutting.
b, c. Nipping or tearing off a polyp or Reinke's edema is incorrect technique.

Hemostasis is usually achieved easily, particularly in benign lesions; the blood is sucked off until bleeding ceases. Blood clots mixed with mucus can be removed simply with a moist cotton wool probe. Even brisk bleeding is usually rapidly controlled by pressure with a pledget of compressed cotton wool on a thread soaked in adrenalin. Almost all bleeding during minor endolaryngeal procedures will cease spontaneously if the surgeon has enough patience. The use of diathermy should be restricted to brisk persistent bleeding. In almost 30 years I have had to pack the larynx only once to achieve hemostasis, and I have had to ligate the superior laryngeal artery twice after arytenoidectomy. It is immaterial whether coagulation is achieved with the laser or with a high-frequency microcoagulator. Both cause burns that obviously heal more poorly and more slowly than smoothly cut wound edges. Furthermore, extensive coagulation leads to marked postoperative perifocal edema, which is rare after simple excision with conventional instruments.

The destruction of polyps, nodules, cysts, or granulomas by the laser reduces the tissue to carbon that can no longer be submitted to histologic examination. This is an unnecessary and time-consuming overkill, attended by delayed wound healing and poor functional results. If a laser is used, it should be employed as a scissors or scalpel for dissection and not for vaporization of tissue.

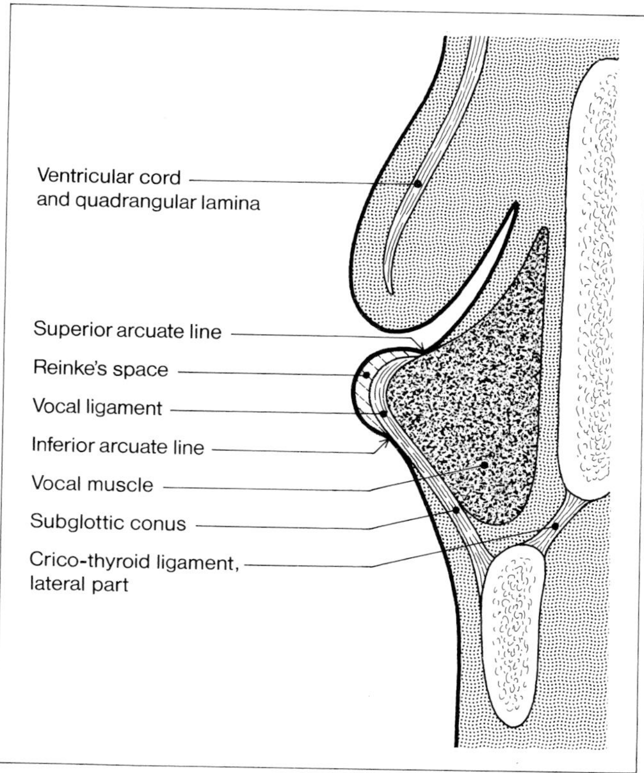

Fig. 32.

Anatomic structures in the main area of interest of endolaryngeal microsurgery.

Surgery that preserves the function of the larynx demands a clear mental picture of the fine anatomical structures and the histopathology of the most important lesions (Figure 32). The area of loose squamous epithelium over the vocal cords is limited by the arcuate lines, the vocal processes, and the anterior commissure.[18] Reinke's space is limited basally by the fascial layer overlying the vocalis muscle, and this fascial layer is thickened at the free edge of the vocal cord to form the vocal ligament; inferiorly it merges into the conus elasticus, and anteriorly into the cricothyroid ligament. The medial boundary of Reinke's space is formed by a thin layer of squamous epithelium lying on a robust basal membrane. An important goal of endolaryngeal operations must be to preserve Reinke's space, which is very important in the fine modulation of the voice. If Reinke's space is not preserved, the regenerating epithelium adheres to the muscle of the vocal cord or to the vocal ligament, a condition compatible with a serviceable voice but not with a voice that is ideal in all parameters.

Polyps, varices, and most nodules are attached only to the squamous epithelium and are freely mobile with it. The small defect remaining after removal of a polyp usually closes rapidly. Vocal cord cysts usually lie beneath the epithelium but are clearly distinct from the vocal ligament and can be enucleated without permanent damage after slitting the epithelium. In contrast, juvenile papillomas derive their connective tissue pedicle and vessels from Reinke's space itself. Removal of these lesions therefore leads much more often to cicatricial obliteration of this space. Even benign keratoma, carcinoma-in-situ, and microinvasive carcinoma can often be resected without destruction of the vocal ligament or the production of a large epithelial defect. In contrast, the greater part of the epithelium must be removed for Reinke's edema. The regenerating epithelium usually adheres closely to the vocal ligament, leading to phonatory immobility that can be shown by stroboscopy. In chronic laryngitis it is technically very difficult to distinguish the vocal ligament from the epithelium, because Reinke's space is filled by fibrous and inflammatory tissue; the regenerating epithelium is tightly bound to the vocal cord.

Lesions such as polyps, nodules, or small cysts adhering to the epithelium should not be grasped directly with a forceps but held at their edge by a mucosal fold. The lesion is then drawn towards the midline and cut off at its base with a scissors. The mucosal defect should be as small as possible and have entirely smooth edges (Figure 33).

Cysts with a diameter greater than 2 mm should be carefully dissected out with a needle or scissors after a longitudinal incision of the mucosa of the vocal cord has been made. The wall of the cyst should be preserved, if possible (Figure 34). Removal of only a part of the covering of the cyst (deroofing) leads rapidly to recurrence.

Various techniques are recommended for Reinke's edema, including scarification, removal of the submucosal mucus by suction (microsuction), removal of a narrow strip of mucosa followed by fixation of the mucosal remnant to the body of the vocal cord with fibrin glue,[44] or even burning holes into the mucosa with the laser. Most often stripping is recommended; This usually leaves irregular lacerated mucosal edges, which become involuted and form protuberances resembling a polyp. The correct technique for Reinke's edema is to draw the edematous mass towards the midline with a small forceps, and then to divide the epithelium sharply and smoothly with small scissors (Figure 35). The edema is most pronounced just in front of the apex of the vocal process of the arytenoid cartilage and becomes less apparent towards the anterior commissure. I prefer to make the first incision about 1 mm medial to the superior arcuate line, followed by a second incision about 1 mm superior to the inferior arcuate line. The incisions run towards each other and end 2 to 3 mm behind the anterior commissure. The edematous mass is now removed in one piece, and any secretion remaining on the surface of the vocal ligament is suctioned off.

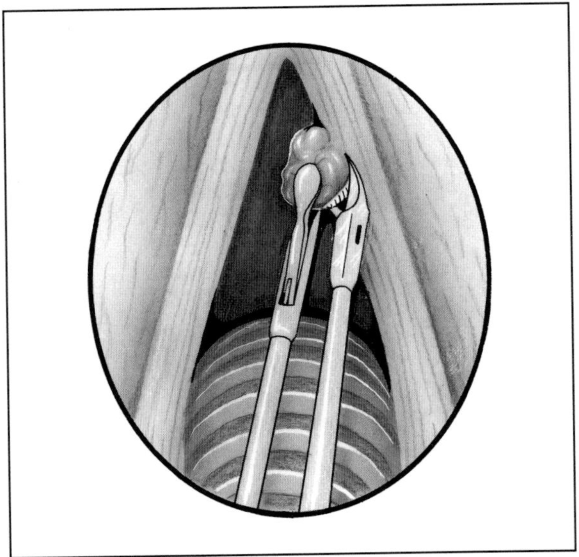

Fig. 33.

Polyps or nodules are removed by drawing the mucosa medially with a small forceps, and the lesion is then excised in one piece with scissors.

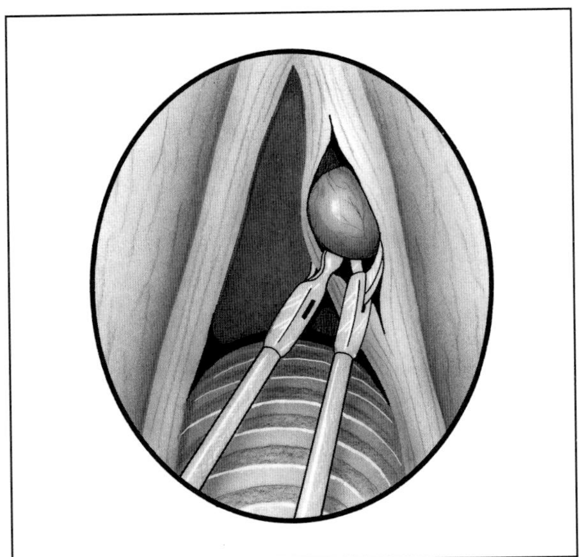

Fig. 34.

Submucosal cysts are dissected bluntly from Reinke's space with a needle or scissors, if possible in one piece, after slitting of the epithelium.

The operation can be carried out in one sitting provided that very great care is taken to ensure that denudation of the anterior commissure or tearing of the mucosa of the anterior commissure does not occur. The patient may complain of prolonged dysphonia or even complete aphonia after bilateral operation at one sitting. Re-epithelialization of a vocal cord requires about 2 months. In pronounced Reinke's edema I now prefer to operate in two stages, because the postoperative dysphonia is usually considerably less. A two-stage procedure and the postoperative recovery period take almost 6 months. An exact operative technique almost always achieves a voice that is satisfactory for everyday use and that will even withstand stress.

A procedure similar to that for Reinke's edema can be used for chronic hyperplastic laryngitis, provided that the space does not show marked inflammatory infiltration and fibrosis (Figure 36). Surgery of advanced chronic laryngitis with epithelial hyperplasia, keratosis, and thick fleshy vocal cords is considerably more difficult because the vocal ligament is difficult to distinguish from the inflammatory infiltrate. Too-deep dissection exposing the vocalis muscle is always followed by a defect of the vocal cord causing postoperative dysphonia. In advanced chronic laryngitis the operation should be carried out in several stages rather than by attempting immediate removal of all the thickened epithelium; only small strips of epithelium and submucosal inflammatory tissue are excised to remodel the outline of the vocal cord (Figure 36). In these cases the anterior commissure must be carefully preserved.

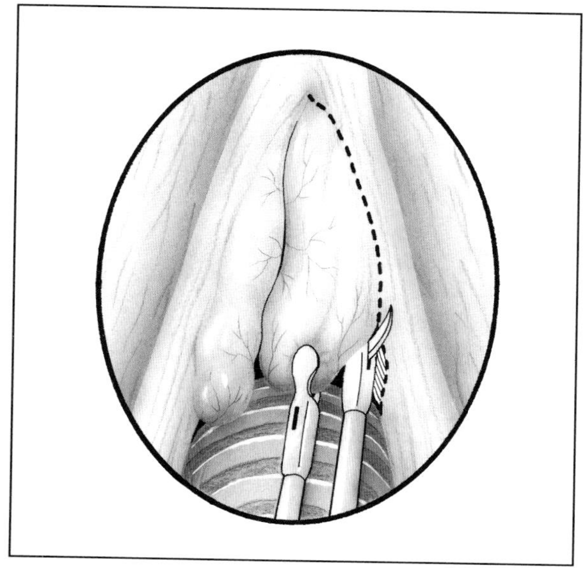

Fig. 35.

Removal of Reinke's edema. The incision is made close to the superior and inferior arcuate lines. The anterior commissure must be carefully preserved.

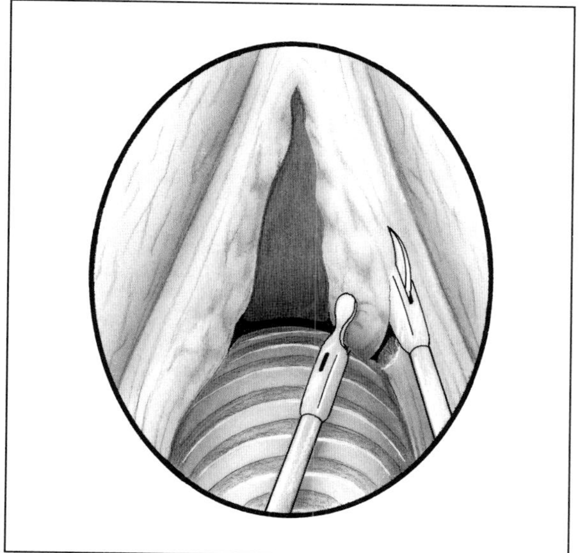

Fig. 36.

Strip excision of a vocal cord for chronic hyperplastic laryngitis. Great care should be taken not to damage the vocal ligament.

Suction coagulation is the usual procedure for the destruction of juvenile papilloma and for the treatment of verrucous acanthosis (Figure 37). The microcoagulator is applied to the papilloma or to the hyperplastic epithelium and the output reduced so that the tissue becomes white and soft rather than burning, so that it can be sucked off easily with little bleeding. The larynx can be quickly and thoroughly cleared by suction coagulation, possibly with division of the pedicle of singular papillomas by the scissors. Local reaction to the coagulation is usually minimal because the action of heat remains strictly localized to the point at which the coagulator is applied.

Biopsies from large tumors are taken with large double forceps. Electrocoagulation may be used liberally in such cases for hemostasis and for debulking of the tumor.

Excision biopsy is routinely used for all small benign or precancerous lesions. An incision is first made round the lesion in apparently healthy tissue, and the lesion is then dissected free from the underlying tissue, in one piece if possible. Benign keratoma, carcinoma-in-situ, and microinvasive carcinoma are freely mobile over the vocal cord and can be removed without damaging the vocal ligament (Figure 38). The vocal ligament and the adjoining superficial muscle fibers are only resected if tumor tissue can be seen lying submucosally on the vocal ligament, thus extending the procedure to a limited endolaryngeal cordectomy.

I only carry out endolaryngeal cordectomy if the lesion is limited to the superficial muscle layers. External access is to be preferred for deeper extension of the tumor into the vocal cord musculature, since it guarantees a good view and the possibility of immediate reconstruction of the vocal cord. A dissecting needle coupled to the high-frequency processor-controlled electrosurgical unit reduces the bleeding during dissection. Excisions of the vestibular fold and of the supraglottic areas do not often follow a routine pattern. The technique of arytenoidectomy is described in the section on paralysis of the recurrent laryngeal nerve (page 90).

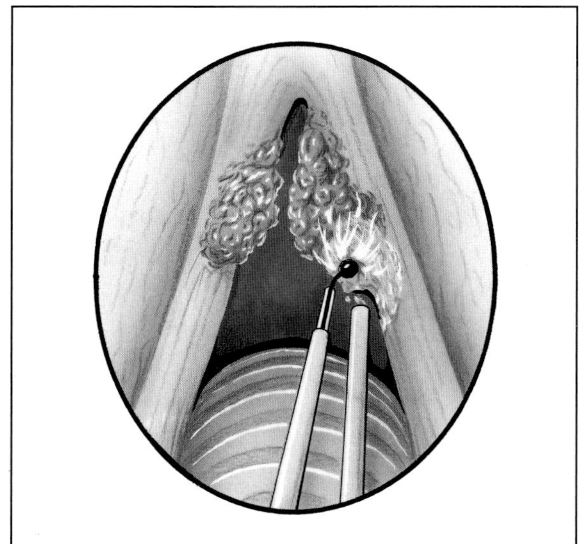

Fig. 37.

Suction coagulation for removal of a juvenile laryngeal papilloma. The papilloma is "parboiled" with a microcoagulator until it becomes white and is then removed by suction.

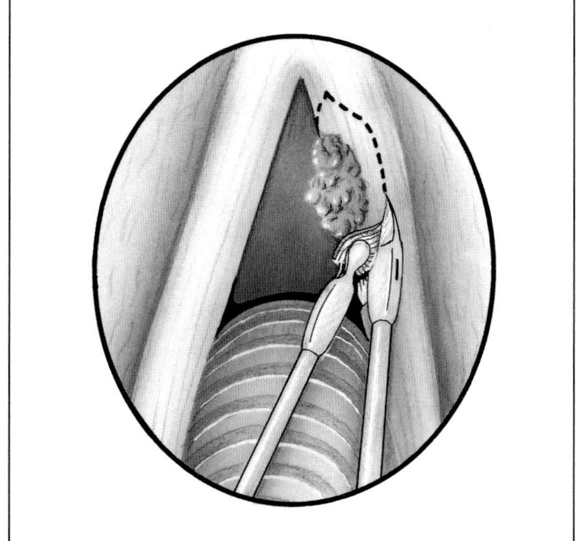

Fig. 38.

Endoscopic excision of a microinvasive carcinoma of the vocal cord. The tumor is circumscribed with scissors and then dissected from the vocal cord. The depth of excision is determined by the depth of infiltration. The tumor should not be resected endoscopically if it has deeply infiltrated the vocal cord musculature. Hemostasis is achieved by microcoagulation.

It is the surgeon's duty to ensure that the surgical specimen or biopsy material is delivered to the pathologist in such a way that the latter can orient himself as to the tissue's site of origin and examine serial sections from the entire specimen.[32] A frequent gross error is to place tissue removed from the vocal cord in formalin solution, in which it retracts and rolls up and then cannot be orientated later. Biopsies taken in this way may produce oblique sections in which it is impossible to decide whether a lesion is preinvasive or invasive and whether the lesion has been completely removed and where its various edges lie. The pathologist is then not to blame if he limits himself to a brief diagnosis without addressing any other question.

We put any tissue removed immediately on a small piece of absorbent cardboard, spread the tissue out, fix it with needles, and write on the cardboard where the front, back, top, and bottom edges lie, so that sections can later be orientated (Figure 39). To this is added a sketch, a statement as to the site from where the tissue was taken, and finally the questions that the pathologist should answer.

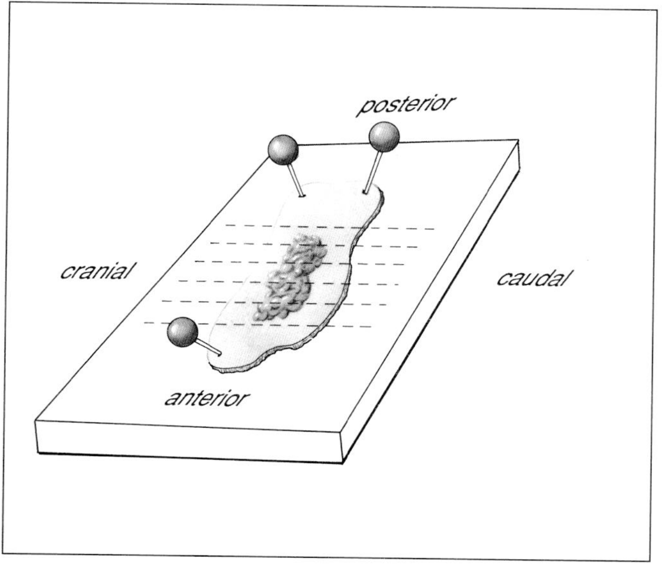

Fig. 39.

Material excised from the larynx must be carefully orientated and fixed to sheets of cardboard. The position of the specimen must be marked on the cardboard before the fixed material is submitted for histologic study.

8. Complications

Because there have been only a few reports of complications of microlaryngoscopy and endolaryngeal microsurgery, they are seldom mentioned.

It is the duty of the anesthesiologist to inform the patient about the anesthesia, whereas the laryngologist must provide details about any possible local damage resulting from the operation. In doubtful cases with a particularly high operative risk the anesthesiologist and the surgeon must decide jointly whether microlaryngoscopy should be carried out, or whether there is a suitable, safer alternative.

The surgeon must warn the anesthesiologist about any expected difficulties with intubation. In such cases an emergency bronchoscope should be available, allowing the laryngologist to ensure an airway in the presence of a rigid obstruction such as a tumor and allowing intubation or tracheotomy to be carried out. In large malignant tumors it is better to carry out a prophylactic tracheotomy than to expose the patient to the risk of unsuccessful intubation. I do not share the frequently expressed fear that tumor particles can be torn off with the endotracheal tube and implanted at other sites.

General complications include circulatory and respiratory disorders resulting from the anesthesia. Indeed several authors have reported myocardial infarction after microlaryngoscopy. I have not seen this myself, but it can never be completely excluded in elderly patients, who often suffer from cardiac disease.

Local injury such as laceration, bruising, or hematoma of the lips or tongue can usually be prevented by careful introduction of the laryngoscope.

The enamel on the edge of the incisors is often splintered if a tooth guard is not used. Furthermore, fracture of the neck of a tooth and loosening or even extraction of individual teeth can happen relatively easily if the patient has periodontal disease or severe caries. Overcrowned teeth and bridges are in particular danger because it is never possible to know how much pressure they will withstand. Both the surgeon and the anesthesiologist should check the patient's teeth after the operation. Injury to the teeth requires immediate examination by a dentist, confirmation of the extent of the injury, and immediate treatment of small lesions.

Tearing and laceration of the palate and of the lateral wall of the pharynx are painful, unpleasant, and sadly all too common. These injuries are caused by the pressure of the laryngoscope on the base of the tongue or the oropharynx and are very difficult to prevent because the elasticity of these tissues is very variable. Many of these injuries are only discovered when the patient complains that he has pain similar to that after tonsillectomy or an external swelling in the neck. Therefore, it should be a rule to inspect these regions carefully after removal of the laryngoscope and to search deliberately for concealed lacerations. Deeper lacerations should be sutured immediately, and antibiotics must be given in all cases to prevent parapharyngeal extension of the infection.

Individual cases of disturbance of taste and paralysis of the lingual and hypoglossal nerves have been reported after microlaryngoscopy, but these problems have usually resolved rapidly and spontaneously. Bleeding from the larynx during or after the operation is seen only after major procedures such as arytenoidectomy or cordectomy. Hemostasis can usually be achieved by adrenaline-soaked pledgets, deliberate coagulation, or sutures, if necessary. Massive bleeding may demand packing of the larynx followed by a laryngotomy or ligation of the superior laryngeal artery.

Postoperative edema is relatively unusual, even after extensive operations, and is usually not marked, but it is more common after the use of the coagulator or the laser. In children we use prophylactic intravenous steroids to prevent edema, for example after the removal of extensive papillomas.

Granulomas, scars, and adhesions can develop after the operation, but they can often be prevented by careful, atraumatic surgery. Patients with a tendency to form hypertrophic scars or keloids are at particular risk and can develop excessive scar tissue in the larynx. The treatment of granulomas and scars after endolaryngeal procedures is dealt with later.

9. Postoperative Care

Many laryngologists recommend a period of absolute voice rest after endolaryngeal microsurgery, but this is difficult to maintain and is ignored by many patients. I have become less rigorous in this respect over the years and now only urge the patient to use his voice sparingly for as long as possible. If he must speak he should do so with a normal voice and must on no account whisper. Coughing and clearing the throat should also be avoided, and singing or shouting forbidden. Coughing should be treated by cough suppressants and mucolytic agents. Normal use of the voice is allowed after the lesion heals.

Antibiotics are given after extensive operations such as arytenoidectomy, and inhalation therapy is advisable in all cases. We advise twice-daily steam inhalations for 20 minutes with dilute aqueous solution of camomile, sage oil, or panthenol. Dry nebulizers, concentrated ether oils, mucosal irritants, drying agents, and cold nebulizers are not recommended.

The patient usually leaves hospital the day after the operation, but voice therapy does not begin until the wound has healed. In many cases of polyps and cysts, the voice returns spontaneously to normal so that further treatment is superfluous. Vocal rehabilitation is always indicated after removal of nodules in women and contact granulomas in men. These lesions can be permanently relieved only by treatment of the underlying functional disorder. Phoniatric procedures are also helpful after removal of Reinke's edema and chronic laryngitis to allow the patient to learn again how to speak with his remodelled vocal cord.

A clear improvement of the voice can often be achieved by voice exercises after resection of the vocal cord or arytenoidectomy.

Postoperative phoniatric procedures have not yet been put on a firm footing, with the result that every speech therapist uses individual relaxation exercises, procedures for strengthening the voice, phonation and breathing exercises, and also possibly stimulation with electric current.[5]

Special Section

1. Statistics

The data on 4663 microlaryngoscopies carried out at the Ear, Nose and Throat Clinic of the University of Marburg from April 1, 1973, to July 31, 1989, were collected by my colleague Dr. W. Schulze (Table 1). They do not include microlaryngoscopies carried out during panendoscopy of the upper and lower respiratory tract. The summary tables provide a rough overview of the material seen at the Marburg Clinic and supplement our earlier statistics and that of other authors.[22, 39]

The number of microlaryngoscopies carried out for adhesions, stenosis, and intubation injuries is particularly remarkable compared with the data in the 2nd edition of this book.

The age distribution of the most important benign vocal cord lesions at the time of first diagnosis is summarized in Table 2.

Table 1. Statistics of microlaryngoscopies carried out at the ENT clinic of the Philipps University, Marburg from April 1, 1973, to July 31,1989.

Diagnosis	Male	Female	No. of Patients	No. of Ops.
Vocal cord polyp	371	137	508	526
Vocal cord nodules	0	104	104	106
Screamers' nodules	16	8	24	24
Ectasia and varix	1	6	7	7
Contact granuloma	137	0	137	146
Cyst	126	117	243	249
Reinke's edema	211	107	318	347
Chronic laryngitis	222	19	241	288
Interarytenoid pachydermia	4	2	6	6
Tuberculosis	9	3	12	13
Sarcoidosis	5	2	7	9
Juvenile papilloma	98	59	157	274
Verrucous acanthosis	16	1	17	30
Amyloid deposits	6	5	11	15
Hyperplasia of the vestibular fold	23	1	24	25
Congenital anomalies	5	6	11	11
Keratosis and keratoma	141	16	157	184
Carcinoma and carcinoma-in-situ of the vocal cord	522	35	557	565
Supraglottic carcinoma	72	7	79	82
Hypopharyngeal carcinoma	81	6	87	94
Misc. tumors	61	36	97	105
Follow-up of tumors	289	32	321	379
Adhesions, stenosis, and intubation injury	254	251	505	805
Paralysis	44	209	253	268
Misc.	61	36	97	105
Total	2775	1205	3980	4663

Table 2. Age distribution at the time of first diagnosis of the most frequent benign lesions of the vocal cords

Diagnosis	0–10	11–20	21–30	31–40	41–50	51–60	61–70	>70
1 Polyp	0	12	98	134	192	91	22	5
2 Cyst	4	10	27	37	50	44	31	21
3 Contact granuloma	0	0	1	23	58	27	0	0
4 Reinke's edema	0	1	9	28	112	119	36	11
5 Chronic laryngitis	0	3	16	45	81	59	33	4
6 Juvenile papilloma	31	19	21	32	29	13	7	1
7 Nodules	0	9	34	39	20	1	1	0

2. Benign Lesions

a. Vocal Cord Polyps (Figures 40–56)

Polyps are by far the most frequent benign vocal cord lesions presenting with hoarseness. They arise only from the membranous part of the vocal cord and not from the cartilaginous part or the supra- or infraglottic regions. No disease of other organs that resembles the vocal cord polyp is known. About 70% of our patients with vocal cord polyps were men, none was younger than 18 years, and most were between 30 and 50 years old. Of all vocal cord polyps 90% were solitary and only about 10% were bilateral or multiple on one side (see Figures 55, 56).

Vocal cord polyps are not true tumors, even if they are often termed fibromas, myxomas, or hemangiomas. They are also not due to an inflammatory process in the strictest sense.

More than 80% of our patients with vocal cord polyps were cigarette smokers, many admitted to habitual or professional vocal abuse, but none was a trained singer.

Histology and electron microscopy have shown that the disease apparently arises from the submucosal capillaries of the vocal cord.[10] Indeed, during microlaryngoscopy a cluster of dilated capillaries forming the nucleus of the angiectatic polyp can sometimes be seen (Figures 40, 41, 42, 43). Blood is often extravasated from the ectatic vessels, and subepithelial hematomas of the vocal cord are also often pronounced. Yellowish discoloration of the vocal cord around the polyp is evidence of previous bleeding (Figure 42). In other cases, the secretion is mainly fibrin, producing a translucent gelatinous type of polyps (Figures 44, 45). These extravasates are organized by sprouting capillaries, like a thrombus. Further bleeding and secretion of fibrin from the new capillaries cause the polyp to grow.[20, 24]

Fig. 40.

Cluster of convoluted vessels covered by thin epithelium on the left vocal cord. This change can be interpreted as the early manifestation of a telangiectatic vocal cord polyp.

Fig. 41.

Telangiectatic polyp on the right vocal cord. To be seen through the thin transparent epithelium is the vascular cluster which represents the nucleus of the polyp.

Fig. 42.

Broad-based, sessile telangiectatic vocal cord polyp. Yellow discoloration of the surrounding mucosa resulting from hemosiderin deposits due to previous submucosal hemorrhage.

Fig. 43.

Large telangiectatic vocal cord polyp hanging in the glottis.

Fig. 44.

Translucent gelatinous vocal cord polyp filled with fibrin.

Fig. 45.

Large gelatinous polyp of the right vocal cord. Unlike Reinke's edema, this lesion affects one side of the larynx only, and only part of the epithelium of the vocal cord is elevated.

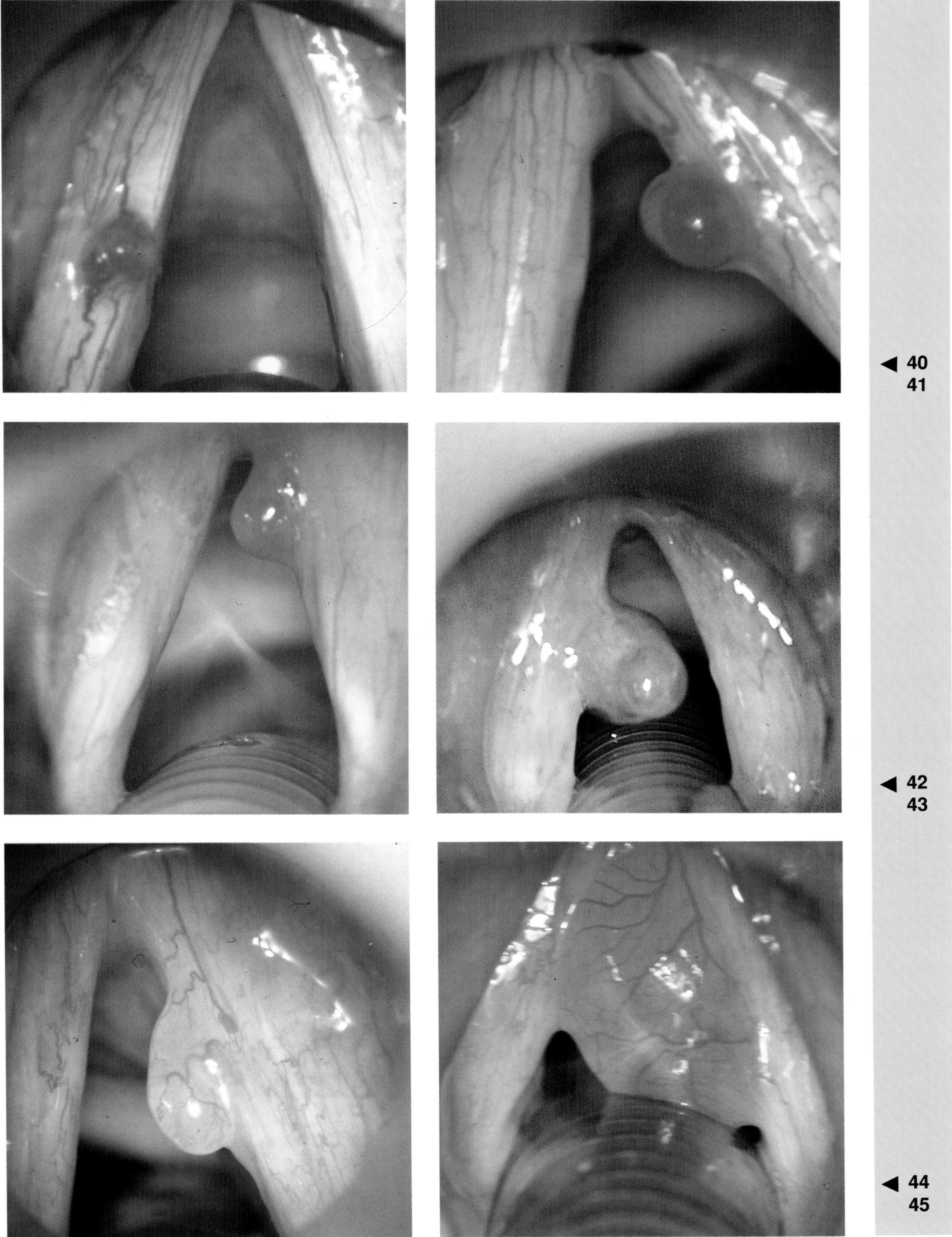

◀ 40
41

◀ 42
43

◀ 44
45

Pathogenetically, all vocal cord polyps – whether purely teleangiectatic, purely gelatinous, or of the predominant mixed type – may be interpreted as being products of phonotrauma.

The squamous epithelium covering the polyp is usually thin and translucent. Some cases show superficial keratinization (Figure 49) and ulcers of mechanical origin with secondary inflammation (Figure 50). A proven relationship between polyps and the development of carcinoma has so far not been published. My own series contains several patients showing a polyp combined with a carcinoma of the opposite cord, chronic laryngitis, Reinke's edema, or a vocal cord cyst.

Polyps arise from the anterior half of the membranous vocal cord and only rarely further posteriorly. Small polyps are difficult to distinguish from a cyst or nodule, even under microlaryngoscopy. In such cases histology confirms the diagnosis by demonstrating the typical nucleus of capillaries which is present in a polyp but absent in a nodule. Large polyps hang in the glottis and can even become impacted, causing attacks of asphyxia. The voice may be normal if the polyp is hanging in the subglottic space, but the patient suddenly becomes hoarse if the polyp impacts in the glottis (Figures 47, 48, 51).

Large polyps often cause contact reactions on the opposite vocal cord, such as pits, epithelial hyperplasia, or circumscribed edema (Figures 52, 53, 54). These contact lesions only need attention if they are too extensive to undergo spontaneous resolution.

Figures 55 and 56 are examples of multiple polyps.

Fig. 46.

Histologic section of this common form of vocal cord polyp shows dilated vessels in the center, fibrin secretion, and fibrous transformation of the nucleus of the polyp.

Fig. 47.

View of a large vocal cord polyp whose surface is partly ulcerated and covered by fibrin due to mechanical irritation.

Fig. 48.

Large mixed pendulous vocal cord polyp hanging in the glottis.

Fig. 49.

Vocal cord polyps occasionally have a keratinized surface.

Fig. 50.

Very large polyp partially ulcerated and covered by fibrin. This appearance closely resembles a granuloma.

Fig. 51.

This polyp had reached such a size that it had already led to choking attacks.

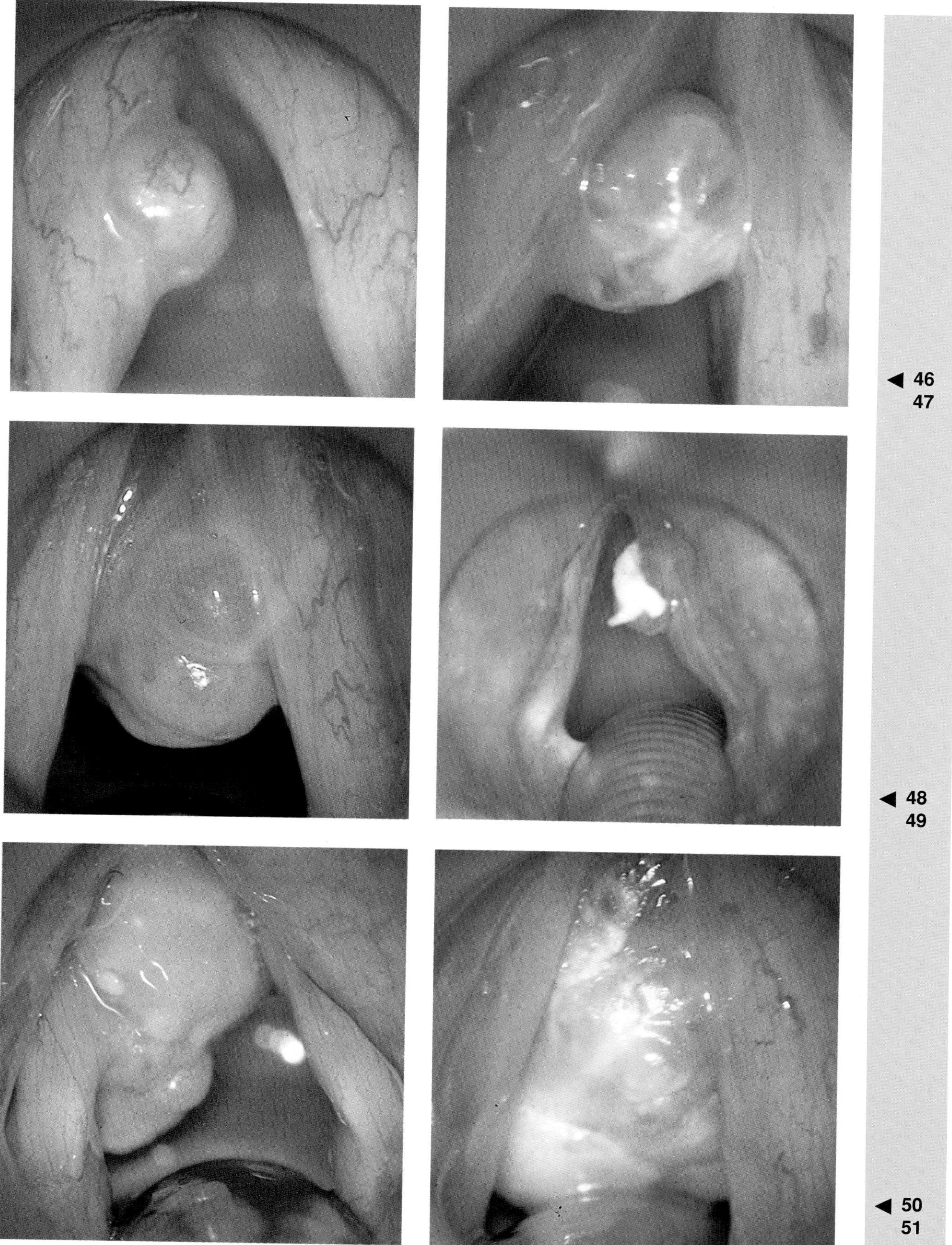

◀ 46
47

◀ 48
49

◀ 50
51

Removal of a polyp with a forceps and scissors takes only a few minutes. The mucosa of the polyp is grasped at its base; the polyp is drawn towards the midline away from the vocal cord and is then cut off with scissors in the correct layer (see Figure 33). Punches, snares, laser, cryosurgery, and the suction biopsy apparatus are completely superfluous for this minor procedure.

The voice often returns to normal immediately after the operation. Healing takes about 14 days and the voice can then be fully used.

I have never seen a recurrence, but a further polyp may arise on the opposite vocal cord later on. Mucosal protuberances requiring a second operation can arise from remnants of incompletely removed polyps. Not correctable are scars which result from a too, deep incision, after which the regenerating epithelium becomes attached to the vocal ligament.

Fig. 52.

Polyp of the left vocal cord with marked contact reaction on the opposite vocal cord.

Fig. 53.

Gelatinous polyp of the right vocal cord with thickened epithelium and keratinization of the left vocal cord at the point of contact.

Fig. 54.

Large vocal cord polyp with reactive changes on both vocal cords, closely resembling Reinke's edema.

Fig. 55.

Polyps on both vocal cords situated near the anterior commissure.

Fig. 56.

A very unusual finding: three vocal cord polyps in one patient.

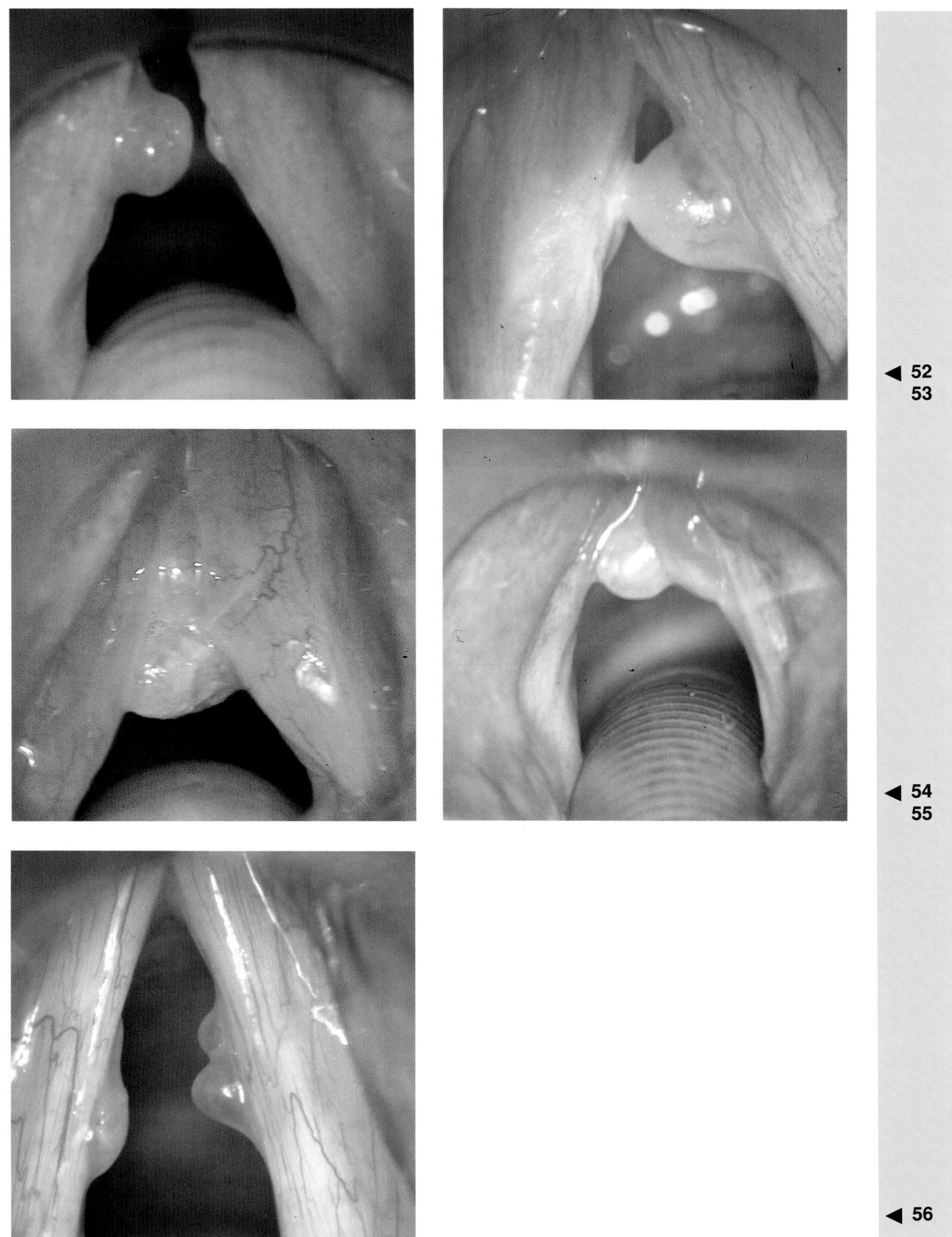

◀ 52
53

◀ 54
55

◀ 56

b. Vocal Cord Nodules (Figures 57–59)

It is not always easy to distinguish a vocal cord nodule from other similar lesions. In my experience true vocal cord nodules develop exclusively in women, usually between the ages of 16 and 45. I have not yet seen a convincing case of a vocal cord nodule in a male.

True nodules are always bilateral lesions arising from the center of the vibrating part of the vocal cord. Small vocal cord nodules present as flat translucent soft mucosal protuberances. If the vocal cord is put under tension during microlaryngoscopy, the small nodules may almost completely disappear (Figure 57). If the nodules are large, they may form two opposing projections that approximate closely when the vocal cords are closed, or one may project into the other (Figure 58). The dome of longstanding hard nodules may even undergo keratinization (Figure 59). Similar unilateral mucosal lesions of the region are not true nodules but are usually small cysts or polyps. The differential diagnosis may be difficult, because cysts or polyps often provoke small mucosal projections as a contact reaction on the opposite vocal cord and then simulate true vocal cord nodules. Accurate differential diagnosis is important because of the prognosis. I have seen many cases of supposed nodules which had been treated for months or even years with voice exercises, but removal of the lesion showed it to be a polyp or a cyst, relieving all vocal problems at a stroke. Thus the diagnosis of a nodule requires both microlaryngoscopy and histologic examination for confirmation. Polyps and cysts can be recognized with certainty by microscopy, but nodules have no characteristic substrate. Occasionally a slightly thickened squamous epithelium is found that is often acanthotic and lies on a very thickened basal membrane. The submucosa of small nodules usually only contains some loose imflammatory cell infiltrate. Older, larger nodules demonstrate a relatively dense circumscribed fibrosis immediately under the basal membrane.

Stroboscopy shows nodules to be the result of functional disorders. Most of these patients are teachers, kindergarten teachers, or mothers who shout at their children. A few of my patients were amateur singers, usually members of choral societies or church choirs, and a few were pop singers, but none had completed proper voice training. The well known term "singers' nodules" is very seldom correct, and the fear of many trained singers of developing nodules is quite groundless. Why these lesions only develop in young women has so far not been explained satisfactorily.

All nodules or suspected nodules should be removed immediately and submitted to histologic study to establish the diagnosis. If the lesion is a cyst or a polyp, treatment is then usually at an end. The operation is a little difficult and should only be carried out by an experienced surgeon using the finest instruments. The nodule is completely removed, leaving a minimal defect in the vocal cord epithelium. Removal of the nodule is followed by voice rest, and speech therapy begins once the lesion has healed. The outlook after excision of a nodule is very good; about 80% of my patients regained a normal voice. Recurrences are possible, requiring a further operation and particularly energetic speech therapy.

c. Screamers' Nodules (Figure 60)

Screamers' nodules are a separate entity from vocal cord nodules. They are underrepresented in my series, because I seldom carry out microlaryngoscopy in these cases. In my own series, screamers' nodules were twice as common in boys as in girls and were found from the fifth year of life until the end of puberty.[55] The children usually have a well developed voice that they use often and to its full capacity. In my view the term "screamers' nodules" is indeed appropriate.

Microlaryngoscopy shows bilateral, symmetrical, flat or spindle-shaped thickenings of the vocal cord with a maximum over the center of the membranous part of the vocal cord. The epithelium over the nodule is often hyperplastic and not translucent. The nodule itself is soft and movable over the underlying tissue (Figure 60).

Fig. 57.

Small, soft vocal cord nodules can be flattened by putting the vocal cords under tension with the laryngoscope.

Fig. 58.

Large vocal cord nodules are often asymmetrical and show a dome on one side and a smooth dent on the other side.

Fig. 59.

Hard vocal cord nodules in cone and crater form.

Fig. 60.

Screamers' nodules in a 9-year-old child. The lesions are more spindle-shaped and extend over the entire length of the membranous part of the vocal cords.

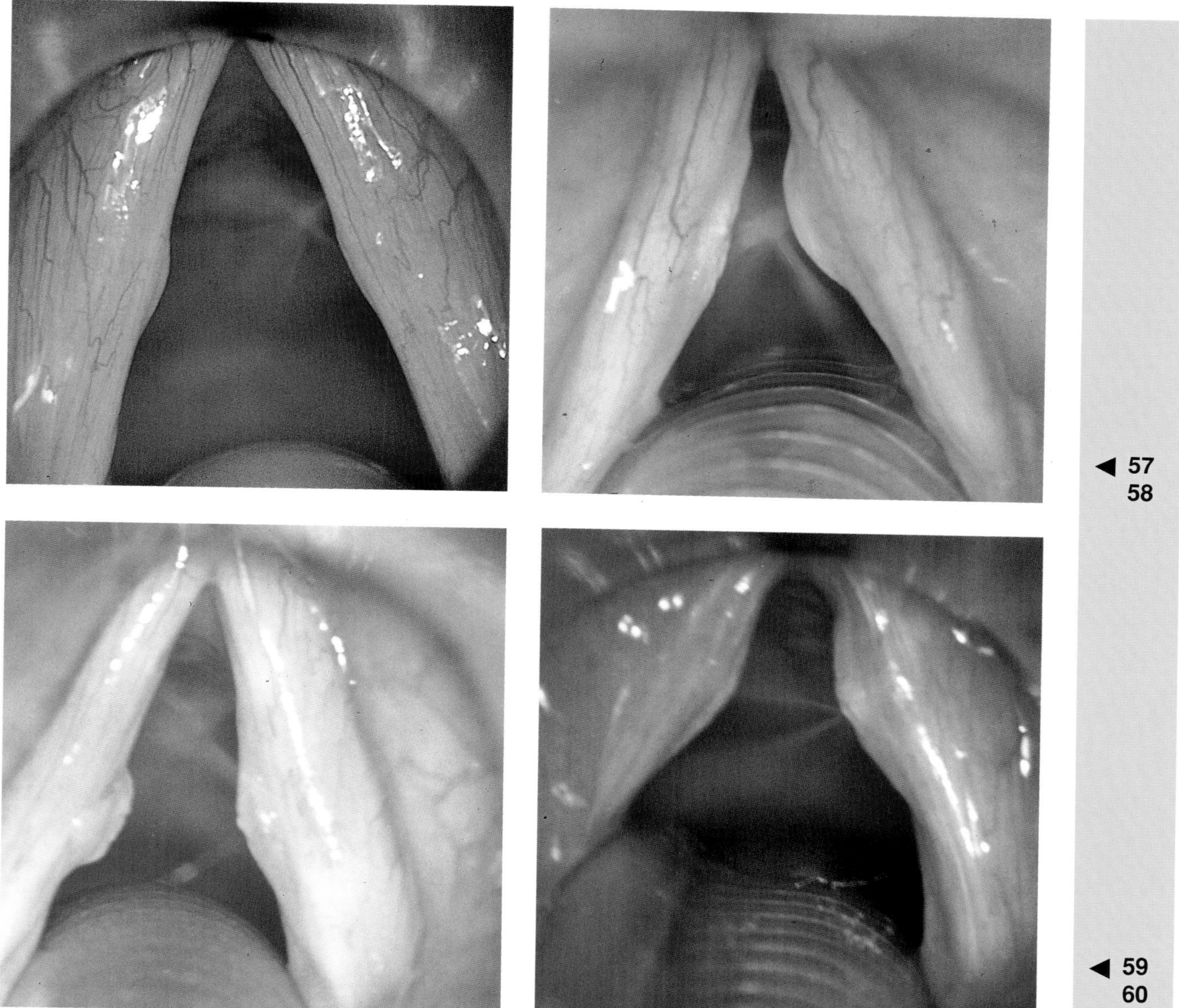

◀ 57
58

◀ 59
60

Screamers' nodules resolve spontaneously when the voice breaks at puberty, and often even earlier. Therefore, our usual plan is simply to advise the parents to encourage their children to use their voices less, but removal of the nodules may be considered if they are very large, if the epithelium is thick, and if the voice is very hoarse.

d. Ectasia and Varices of the Vocal Cord (Figures 61–65)

Varicose dilatation of the vocal cord capillaries is a relatively unusual disease of women. All our patients were subject to considerable vocal strain, and most were trained professional singers. It appears that the state of filling of the dilated capillaries varies with the demands on the voice, because vocal disorders often only appear after a long period of singing. It has repeatedly been reported that the patient may suddenly become aphonic due to a submucous hemorrhage, apparently arising from a ruptured varix that makes further singing impossible.[1, 8]

Half of microvarices affect one vocal cord only, and the rest affect both cords (Figures 61, 62). Examination shows either (1) a vesicular dilatation arising from an individual thickened capillary, often on the free edge of the vocal cord or on its superior surface (Figures 63, 64), or (2) several unusual tortuous and irregular ectatic vessels. A combination of nodules and varices on the vocal cord is less common (Figure 65).

Large varices are excised with scissors after dividing the epithelium, whereas smaller lesions should be coagulated carefully with a needle. The remaining lesion should be as small as possible. So far we have not seen any recurrences. An operation should not be carried out during the acute phase of bleeding into the vocal cord but should be delayed until the blood has been resorbed and the capillary ectasia is clearly visible.

Fig. 61.

Irregular vascular ectasia on a vocal cord of an opera singer.

Fig. 62.

Bilateral vascular ectasia in a singer.

Fig. 63.

Vesicular varicose vascular ectasia on the right cord.

Fig. 64.

Solitary vascular ectasia on the right vocal cord receiving its blood supply posteriorly.

Fig. 65.

Dilated varicose vessels on both vocal cords coincident with evidence of vocal cord nodules.

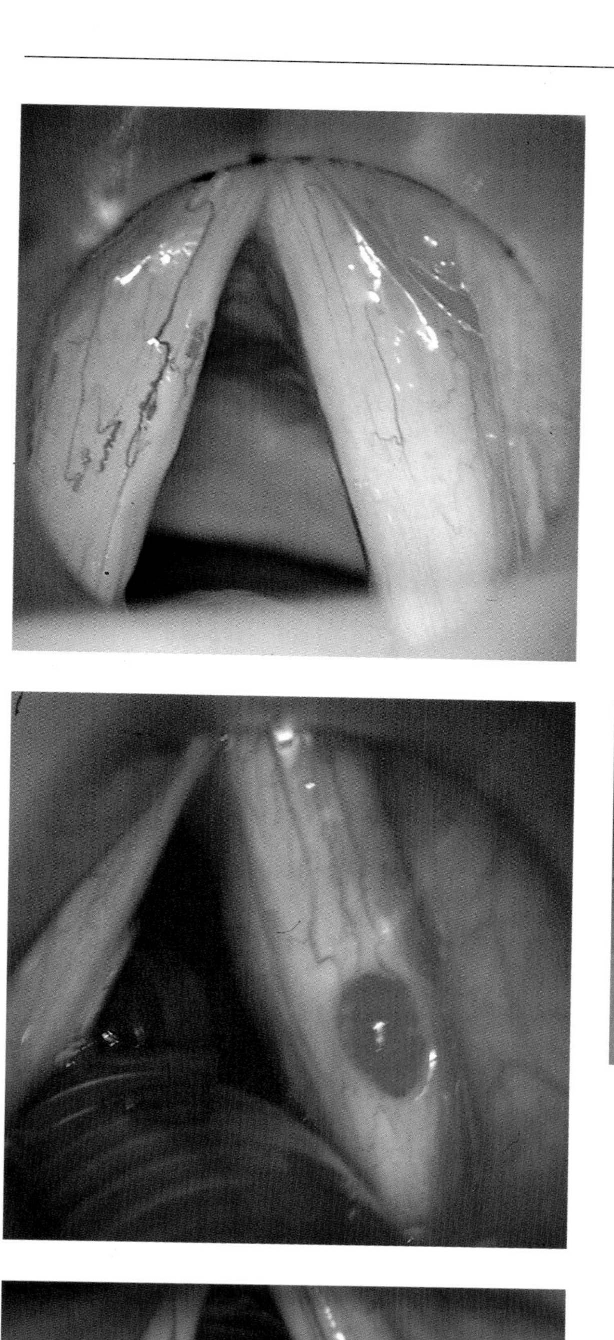

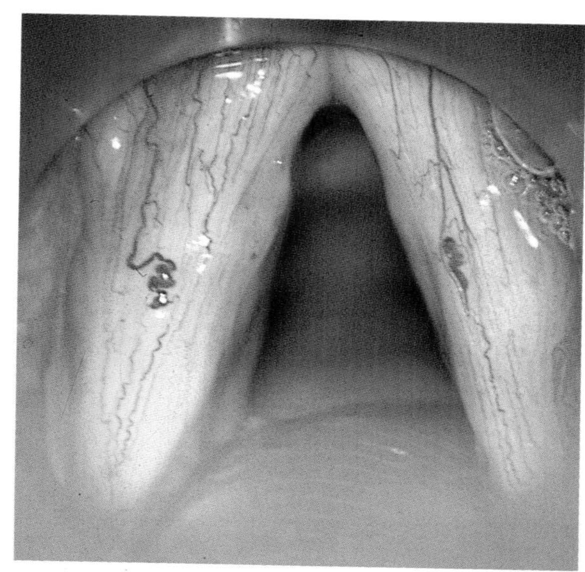

◀ 61
62

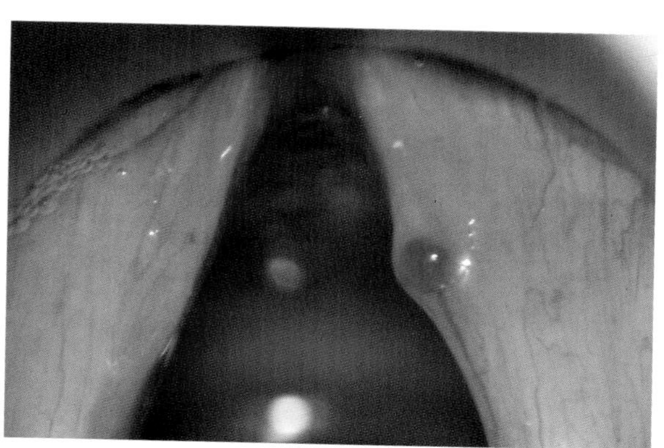

◀ 63
64

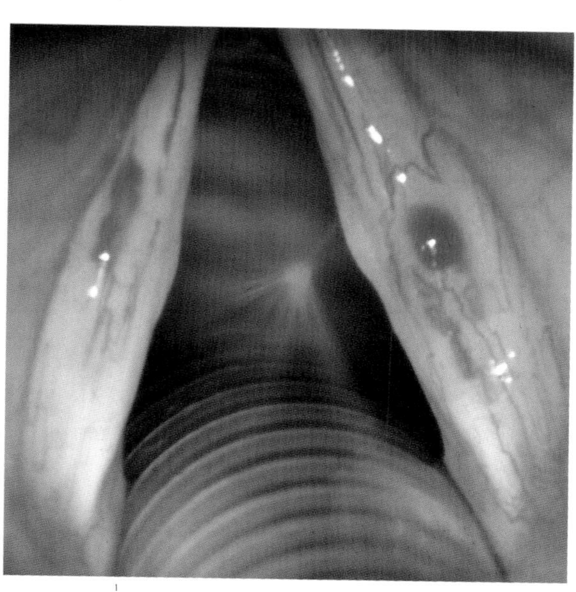

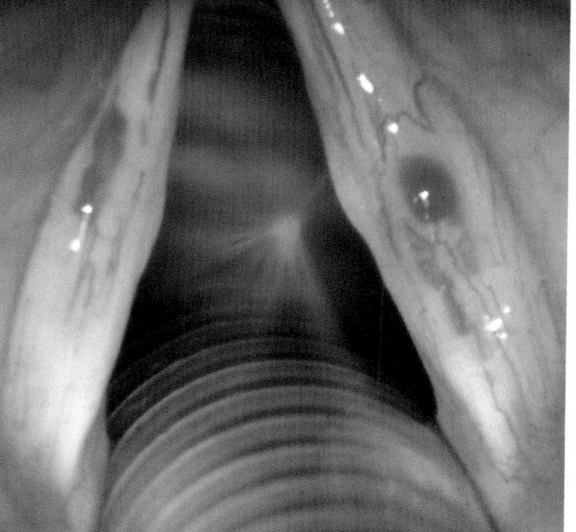

◀ 65

e. Contact Granuloma (Figures 66–72)

Contact granulomas are relatively frequent in our series, exclusively affecting men between the ages of 30 and 60; no patient was younger than 28 and none older than 60.

The lesion was first described by Virchow as a "patellate pachydermia", and was later termed "contact ulcer" by Jackson. It can arise after a single incident of excessive voice use and then usually resolves spontaneously, but in most cases the disease begins insidiously. It is remarkable that these patients tend to speak with a low-pitched, "far back" voice, often slightly retracting the chin. Obsessive clearing of the throat and slight coughing are likewise often heard. Most patients seem to be full of inner tension. They complain of laryngeal discomfort, sometimes also of slight pain radiating to the ear, or foreign body sensations in the throat. Some blood may occasionally be coughed up if part of the granuloma becomes detached and is expelled. It is not uncommon to hear that these men, who are undergoing the so-called "midlife crisis," have marital and/or familial problems. Sometimes the problems underlying the disease are of an occupational or economic nature. In none of our patients was gastroesophageal reflux the causative factor.

If a psychosomatically determined disorder of the larynx does in fact exist, then it is in most cases contact granuloma. I have rarely seen granuloma in trumpeters and clarinettists; in two patients contact granuloma arose secondary to intensive voice exercises after unilateral vocal cord paresis and after cordectomy.

Contact granuloma is always unilateral. Stroboscopy shows clearly how the vocal processes strike each other firmly on phonation, whereas the membranous part of the vocal cord is not taut, so that a narrow cleft remains on phonation. In the early stages a rough area can be seen over the vocal process of one cord, but nothing abnormal is to be seen on the opposite cord. In more advanced cases a granuloma forms with an upper and lower lip that grasp the edges of the opposite vocal process during phonation. Fresh contact granulomas are partially covered by fibrin and are epithelialized only at the edges. Healed contact granulomas appear as thickened epithelial swellings that often even keratinize (Figures 66–72). Histologic examination shows the characteristics of a pyogenic granuloma partially covered by thickened squamous epithelium. Combination with or transition to a carcinoma has not so far been described in this disease.

Most of the patients belong to the upper and middle social classes and are usually very receptive to explanation. The granuloma can resolve spontaneously after thorough explanation of the cause; the patients have then learned to speak with the voice at a higher tone in a more relaxed manner and more forward in the throat and have recognized the relation between their psychological stress and the development of granuloma. Indeed several speech therapists recommend doing nothing, because these granulomas are thought to resolve spontaneously within 2 years.

However, I have seen several patients who suffered recurrent granulomas for more than 10 years, so that I now prefer immediate removal of the granuloma followed by speech therapy and if necessary psychotherapy.

We have had a good primary result with this procedure in 72% of cases, but sadly 28% suffered a recurrence during which a new contact granuloma arose, sometimes within 2 or 3 weeks. In these cases a second or third operation sometimes succeeds, but in a few patients (about 20%) all surgical procedures are in vain. The only thing to do for these patients is to console them that this lesion is bothersome but harmless and never becomes malignant.

Fig. 66.

Early contact granuloma of the right vocal cord showing two smooth granulation tissue bulges over the vocal process.

Fig. 67.

Well-developed contact granuloma of the right vocal cord.

Fig. 68.

Small contact granuloma of the left vocal cord showing the bilabial shape.

Fig. 69.

Large contact granuloma on the right side with a thick "lower lip" and a narrow "upper lip."

Fig. 70.

This case shows very clearly how the contact granuloma arising on the left vocal process grasps the right vocal process during phonation.

Fig. 71.

Healing contact granuloma with superficial keratinization.

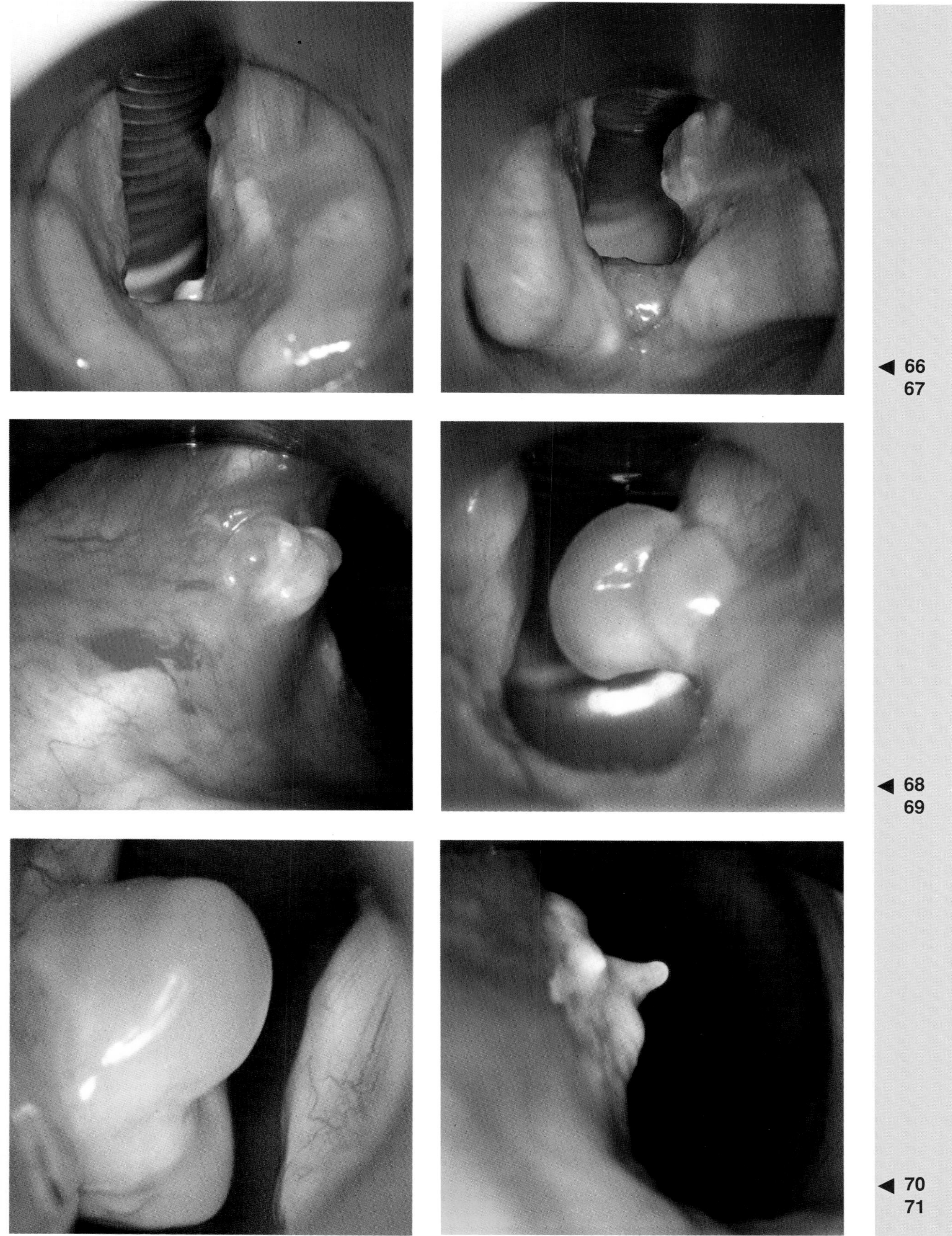

◀ 66
67

◀ 68
69

◀ 70
71

The operation consists of removal of the upper and lower lip of the granuloma with a scissors and effecting hemostasis with by microcautery. I have never had any success with injection of steroids into the area, and furthermore this injection may be followed by cartilage necrosis.

f. Cysts (Figures 73–82)

1. Vocal Cord Cysts

Vocal cord cysts mainly afflict young adults, the average age being 43 years; 6% of my patients were younger than 20 years. There is no clear sex differential.

Two-thirds of vocal cord cysts are lined by squamous epithelium, whereas one-third are lined by cuboidal or columnar epithelium resembling respiratory epithelium. Squamous epithelium, cuboidal epithelium, and columnar epithelium are also often found together. The content of the cyst depends on the lining; it may be watery thin and mucoid, or yellow and inspissated in cysts lined by squamous epithelium. These cysts always lie in Reinke's space immediately beneath the squamous epithelium and rarely within the musculature of the vocal cords.[43] The development of a cyst is dependent on displacement of epithelium into Reinke's space, which is normally free of mucous glands. Cysts lined by columnar or cuboidal epithelium could be due to retention in an endpiece of a seromucinous gland lying in the subglottic surface of the vocal cord.

Vocal cord cysts are mainly unilocular and unilateral, but multilocular and bilateral multiple vocal cord cysts of various sizes are occasionally seen (see Figures 81, 82).

Small vocal cord cysts 1 to 2 mm in diameter are often difficult to distinguish from small polyps or nodules by indirect laryngoscopy, by the laryngeal telescope, and even by microlaryngoscopy. The sac of the cyst can only be recognized after incision of the mucosa (Figures 73, 74, 75). Large vocal cord cysts have a characteristic yellow appearance due to their content of keratin debris (Figures 76–80). Collateral reactive edema and contralateral reactive thickening of the epithelium can also occur in cysts.

Fig. 72.

Older contact callus. Deposit of keratin lies at the site of the granuloma on the left side. On the right side is a keel-shaped projecting vocal process covered by thickened epithelium.

Fig. 73.

Small vocal cord cyst on the left side. This lesion can only be distinguished from a polyp by histologic examination.

Fig. 74.

Small vocal cord cyst on the left side and contact reaction on the right side. Slight yellowish discoloration in the region of the cyst on the left side can be seen. This lesion cannot be distinguished from a vocal cord nodule by indirect laryngoscopy.

Fig. 75.

Small vocal cord cyst on the right side. The cyst lying in Reinke's space is easy to diagnose because of its yellow color.

Fig. 76.

An epidermoid cyst filled with keratinous debris on the free edge of the left vocal cord.

Fig. 77.

The cyst lying in Reinke's space can now be dissected out in one piece after splitting of the mucosa.

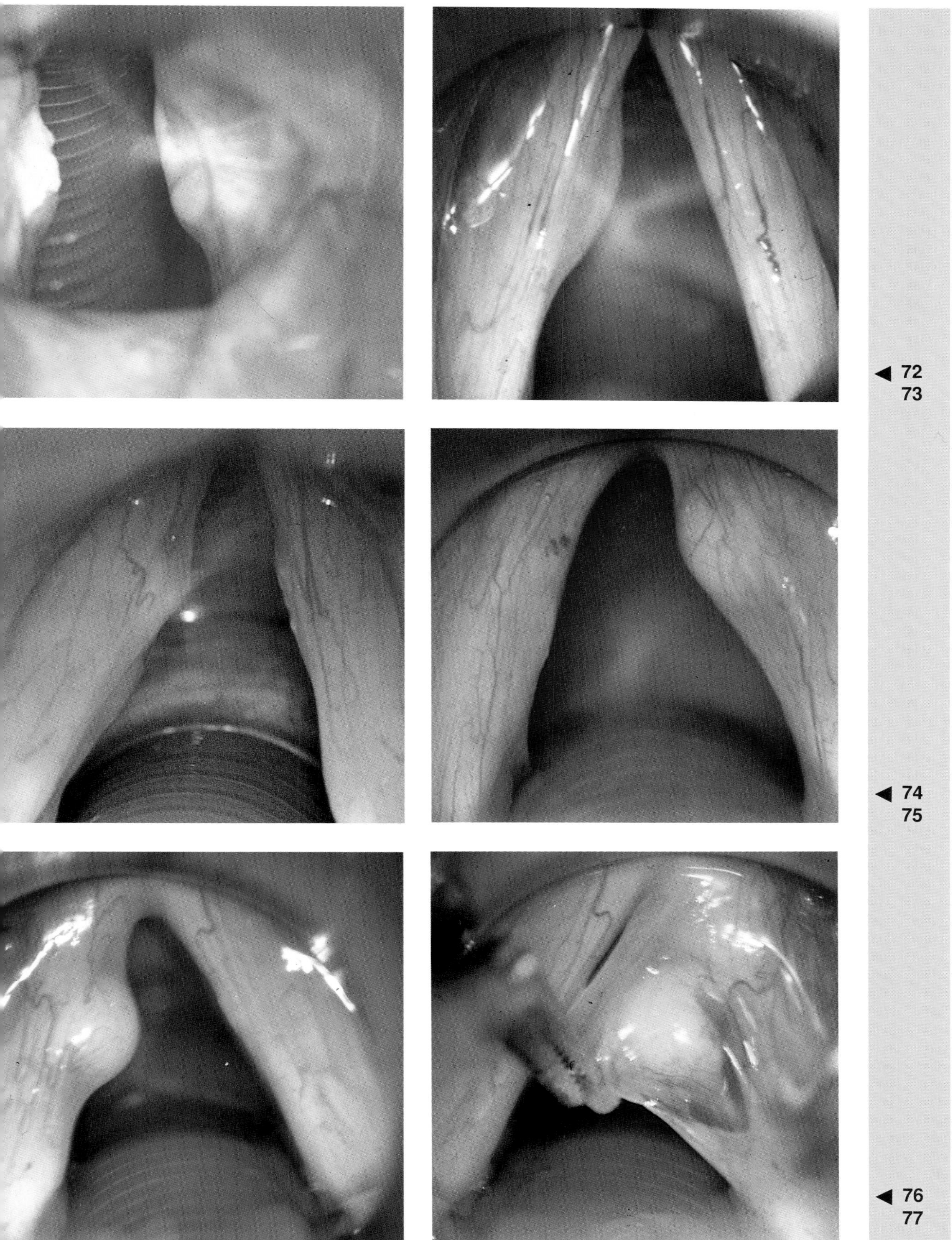

◀ 72
73

◀ 74
75

◀ 76
77

Small cysts 1 mm to 2 mm in diameter can be cleanly separated from the vocal cord together with the overlying epithelium using a curved scissors. If the cyst is larger, it is advisable to incise the mucosa and then remove the sac of the cyst, if possible in one piece, using small scissors or a dissecting needle (Figure 77). Because the wall of the cyst is often fairly thin, it is easily torn, and in these cases it is important to remove the entire cyst wall carefully. Deroofing leads rapidly to recurrence, but I have never seen a recurrence if the sac is removed completely. Postoperative speech therapy is usually not necessary.

2. Solitary Vestibular Fold Cysts (Figures 83–86)

Vestibular fold cysts are equally common in the two sexes, but the average age of 63 years is considerably higher than in the case of vocal cord cysts. However, vestibular fold cysts are occasionally found in children.

Vestibular fold cysts are retention cysts arising in the duct system of the seromucinous glands. Therefore the lining epithelium is of the cuboidal secreting glandular type. A few of these cysts are lined by oncocytes. Cuboidal epithelium may also coexist with various stages of transition to eosinophil granulated oncocytes.

Most vestibular fold cysts have a typical clinical appearance. They project from the ventricle and arise on the lateral wall of the vestibular fold in the depth of the ventricle (Figures 83–86). Less commonly, solitary vestibular fold cysts cause a smooth swelling of the free edge of the fold.

These cysts are usually easy to remove; the cyst is drawn towards the midline until its pedicle can be recognized and cut off. I have never yet seen a recurrence.

Postoperative speech therapy is usually not necessary.

Fig. 78.

Large vocal cord cyst with typical yellowish color on the left side.

Fig. 79.

Large vocal cord cyst on the left side. The capillaries lying over the vocal cord are considerably thickened and tortuous.

Fig. 80.

Very large vocal cord cyst occupying almost half of the membranous part of the left vocal cord.

Fig. 81.

Bilocular vocal cord cyst on the subglottic surface of the right vocal cord.

Fig. 82.

Two vocal cord cysts on the left side and a large cyst on the right side, an unusual finding.

Fig. 83.

Typical vestibular fold cyst prolapsing out of the ventricle.

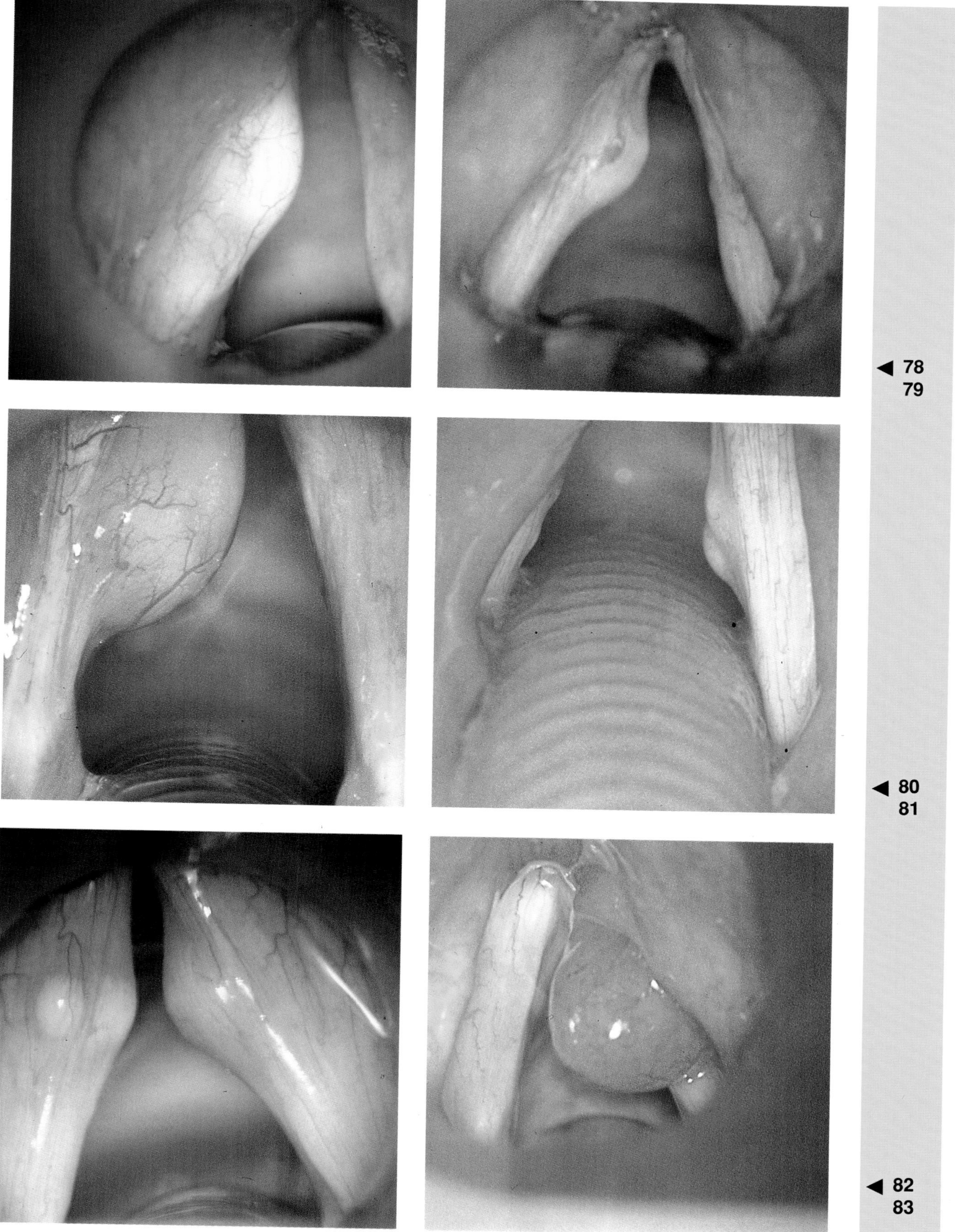

◀ 78
79

◀ 80
81

◀ 82
83

3. Cystic Dysplasia of the Vestibular Fold (Figures 87–90)

Cystic dysplasia of the vestibular fold is characterized by multiple, usually bilateral, multilocular cystic lesions arising from the mucosal glands and presenting as swelling of both vestibular folds (Figures 87–89). In a few cases the lesion may extend over the arytenoid or even into the piriform sinus and then resembles the very rare congenital cyst of this region (Figure 90).[2] Many of these cases are falsely diagnosed as an internal laryngocele.

Incision of the mucosa reveals a system of hollow spaces varying in size that must be dissected out patiently, carefully, and, if possible, completely, using the scissors. At the end of the operation the vestibular fold appears flaccid and empty. The incision should be closed with a few sutures, and the wound surface covered with mucosa.

Fig. 84.

Large oncocytic cyst of the vestibular fold hanging from the ventricle into the glottis.

Fig. 85.

Isolated cyst on the free edge of the vestibular fold lying deeply in the tissue of the fold.

Fig. 86.

Large vestibular fold cyst protruding from the ventricle, with a further small cyst lying on the free edge of the left vestibular fold.

Fig. 87.

Extensive cystic dysplasia of both vestibular folds. On the left side one of the cysts has been opened and viscous gray mucus can be seen draining from it.

Fig. 88.

Extensive bilateral retention cysts in cystic dysplasia of the vestibular folds.

Fig. 89.

In this case the vestibular fold cysts are so extensive that the glottis is completely covered.

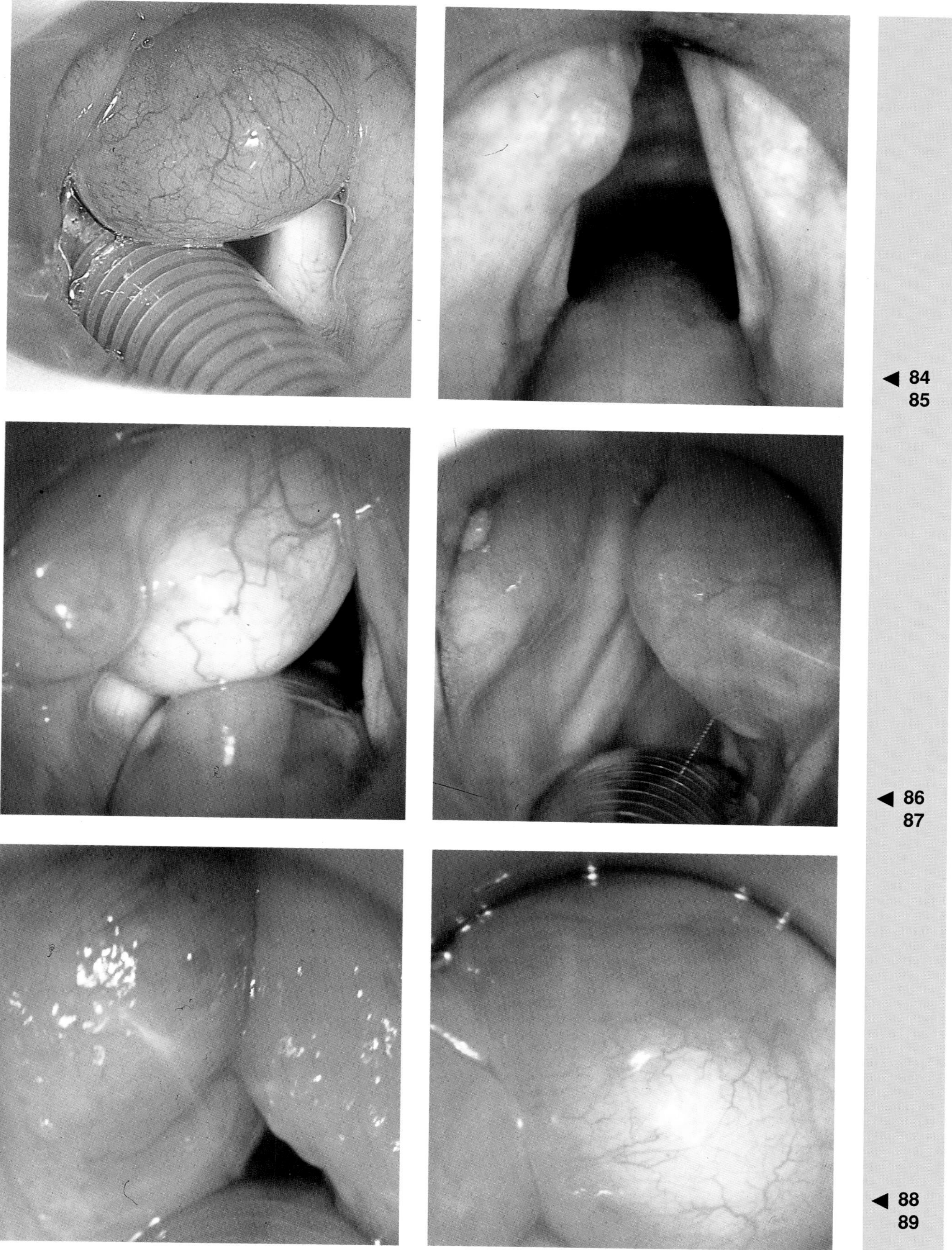

◀ 84
85

◀ 86
87

◀ 88
89

4. Epiglottic Cysts (Figures 91–94)

Epiglottic cysts always arise on the lingual surface of the epiglottis, usually close to the midline. In many cases they extend into the pharyngoepiglottic or aryepiglottic folds.

Epiglottic cysts arise twice as commonly in men as in women, and the average age is about 50 years.

Epiglottic cysts are usually single but may occasionally be multiple (Figure 94). Small epiglottic cysts discovered incidentally need no treatment (Figure 91). Only large cysts displacing the epiglottis and causing dysphagia require treatment (Figures 92, 93). Occasionally the cyst undergoes secondary infection and then simulates an epiglottic abscess. The clinical and microlaryngoscopic appearance is very characteristic, showing a network of vessels over the plump yellow cyst. Many epiglottic cysts are so large that they can scarcely be drawn into a largecaliber laryngoscope. Because of the dense vascular network, excision of these cysts quite often causes bleeding that is not always easy to control by coagulation diathermy. The cyst should be removed in one piece and without opening it, if possible. After the operation the patient often complains of pain similar to that after tonsillectomy.

Most epiglottic cysts are lined by squamous epithelium and a few by a columnar epithelium; rarely oncocytes are found in the wall. To date the pathogenesis of epiglottic cysts has not been explained satisfactorily.

5. Traumatic Cysts (Figure 95)

Traumatic laryngeal cysts follow endotracheal intubation or endolaryngeal surgery. Small cysts over the vocal process or in the interarytenoid region can follow intubation anesthesia. Traumatic cysts lying in the subglottic space beneath the anterior commissure are very rare.

Vocal cord cysts very rarely follow an operation and are caused by the displacement of islands of squamous epithelium into the depth of the cord.

Fig. 90.

The entire left vestibular fold is filled by cysts extending beyond the larynx over the aryepiglottic fold. Multiple cysts are also present in the right vestibular fold.

Fig. 91.

A small cyst on the lingual surface of the epiglottis showing some drainage of its content.

Fig. 92.

Epiglottic cyst almost filling the right vallecula, with a dense vascular network on its surface.

Fig. 93.

Large cyst pedicled on the lingual surface of the epiglottis displacing the epiglottis posteriorly.

Fig. 94.

Two cysts of the lingual surface of the epiglottis displacing the epiglottis posteriorly.

Fig. 95.

A traumatic cyst arising over the apex of the vocal process after intubation.

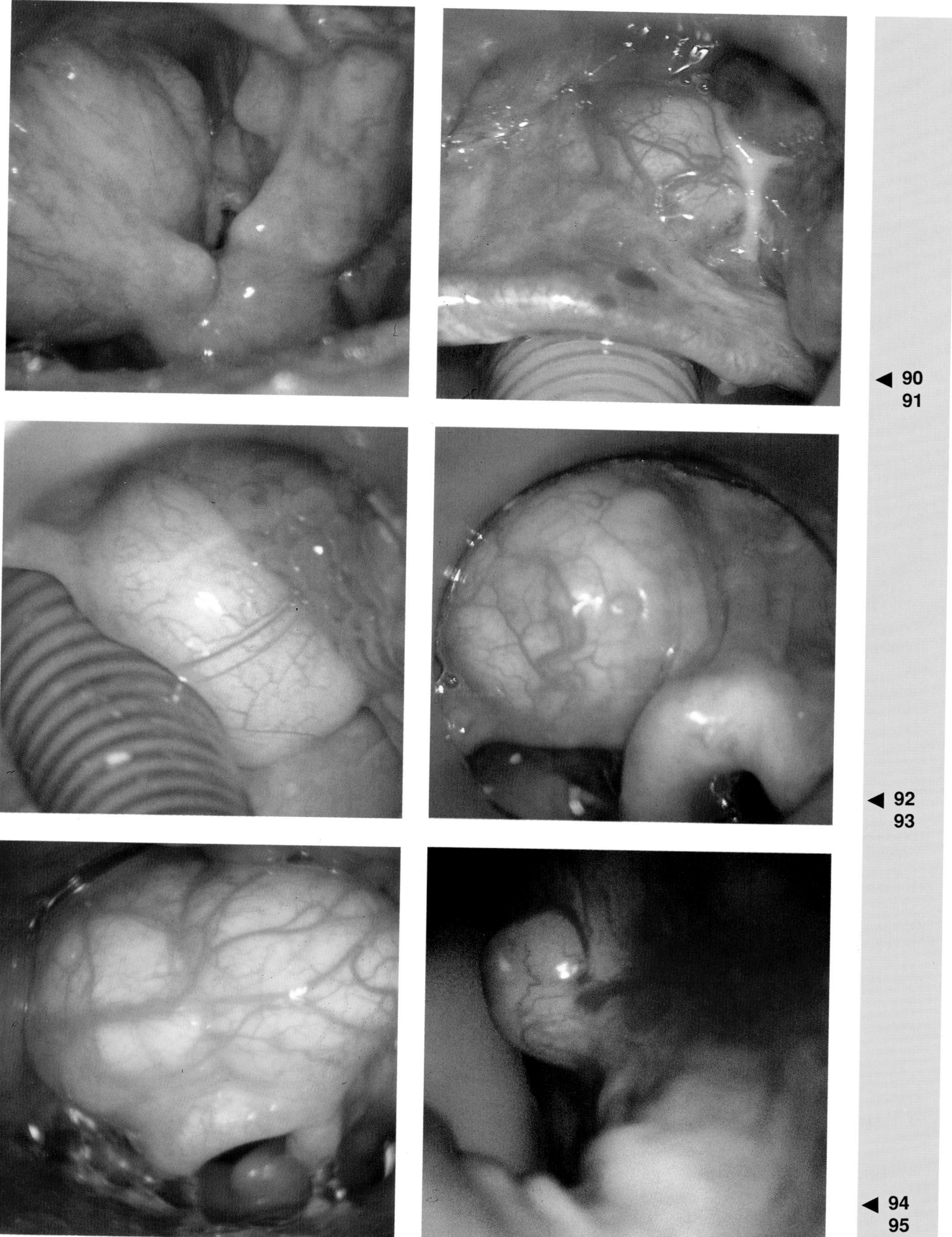

◀ 90
91

◀ 92
93

◀ 94
95

g. Reinke's Edema (Figures 96–102)

Hajek proposed that this relatively frequent disease should be named after the anatomist Reinke, who was the first to investigate the fine anatomical detail of the vocal cord. He described the loose subepithelial mobile layer in the vocal cords which is limited above by the superior arcuate line and below by the inferior arcuate line at the junction of cylindrical and squamous epithelium. The lesion is also termed polypoid corditis, polypoid degeneration, or "laryngite chronique hypertrophic d'aspect pseudomyxomateux" in the French literature.

My own series contain 221 men and 107 women, and the lesion is unusual before the age of 40.

Reinke's edema bears no relation to vocal cord polyps. The most important pathogenetic factor is smoking; 98% of all patients in my series were cigarette smokers. Apart from above average vocal stress, many of these patients showed no other pathogenetic factors such as sinusitis or infection of the upper respiratory tract.[(11)]

Histologic examination shows a gelatinous fluid in a fine honeycomb network beneath a normal vocal cord squamous epithelium.[49] In the early stages the secretion is clear and relatively thin, but in more longstanding cases the secretion is viscous and yellowish, macroscopically resembling that of a glue ear.

The microlaryngoscopic appearance is very characteristic: both vocal cords are always affected, but often to a different degree (Figures 97–99). The early stage consists of a spindle-shaped swelling of the vocal cord extending from the anterior commissure to the apex of the vocal process (Figure 96). Later thick swellings appear, which can be translucent (Figure 98).

The cushions of edema are often so large that they cannot both be accommodated within the glottic cleft and one tends to lie upon the other (Figures 100, 101). Fine areas of keratosis (Figure 99) or shallow epithelial defects covered with fibrin appear in some cases at the point where the edematous swellings rub against each other.

Reinke's edema causes a deep, rough voice with a fairly characteristic sound, and many patients are no longer able to phonate with the glottis. Extensive cases are often complicated by the development of vestibular fold hyperplasia and dysphonia plica ventricularis.

Reinke's edema is certainly not a premalignant condition, but in rare cases it can coexist, precede, or follow carcinoma of the vocal cord. There are no means of telling whether the edema is a reaction to the carcinoma or whether the two have a common genesis in cigarette smoking. Other reactive forms of edema strongly resembling Reinke's edema are occasionally found accompanying polyps or cysts. Sometimes a similar edema arises in patients with vocal cord paralysis.

In my experience Reinke's edema does not respond to cessation of smoking or speech therapy. Puncturing the swelling or sucking off the fluid is usually inadequate because of the loculation of the submucosal space. Refixing the mucosa with tissue glue after sucking off the fluid used to be recommended, but even then the mobile Reinke's space is obliterated to some extent. The most effective method is removal of the excess epithelium together with the mucus, an operation often termed stripping. This description is confusing because it is incorrect to grasp the epithelium with a small forceps and simply strip it from the vocal cord. The correct technique is to elevate the edematous swelling and cut it off smoothly at the supra – and infraglottic boundary between the squamous and respiratory epithelium. To prevent the forma-

Fig. 96.

Early stage of Reinke's edema: the vocal cord epithelium is elevated due to a collection of fluid in Reinke's space and begins to form a swelling.

Fig. 97.

Asymmetrical Reinke's edema: on the right side a thick edematous swelling has already formed, and edema is also beginning to develop on the left side.

Fig. 98.

More advanced stage of Reinke's edema.

Fig. 99.

Asymmetrical Reinke's edema: on the left vocal cord the epithelium begins to thicken due to reactive change.

Fig. 100.

Fully developed Reinke's edema: the cushions of edema are now too big to be accommodated in the larynx and partially overlap each other.

Fig. 101.

Advanced Reinke's edema: the glottis is filled by the edematous swelling, and the patient has respiratory obstruction.

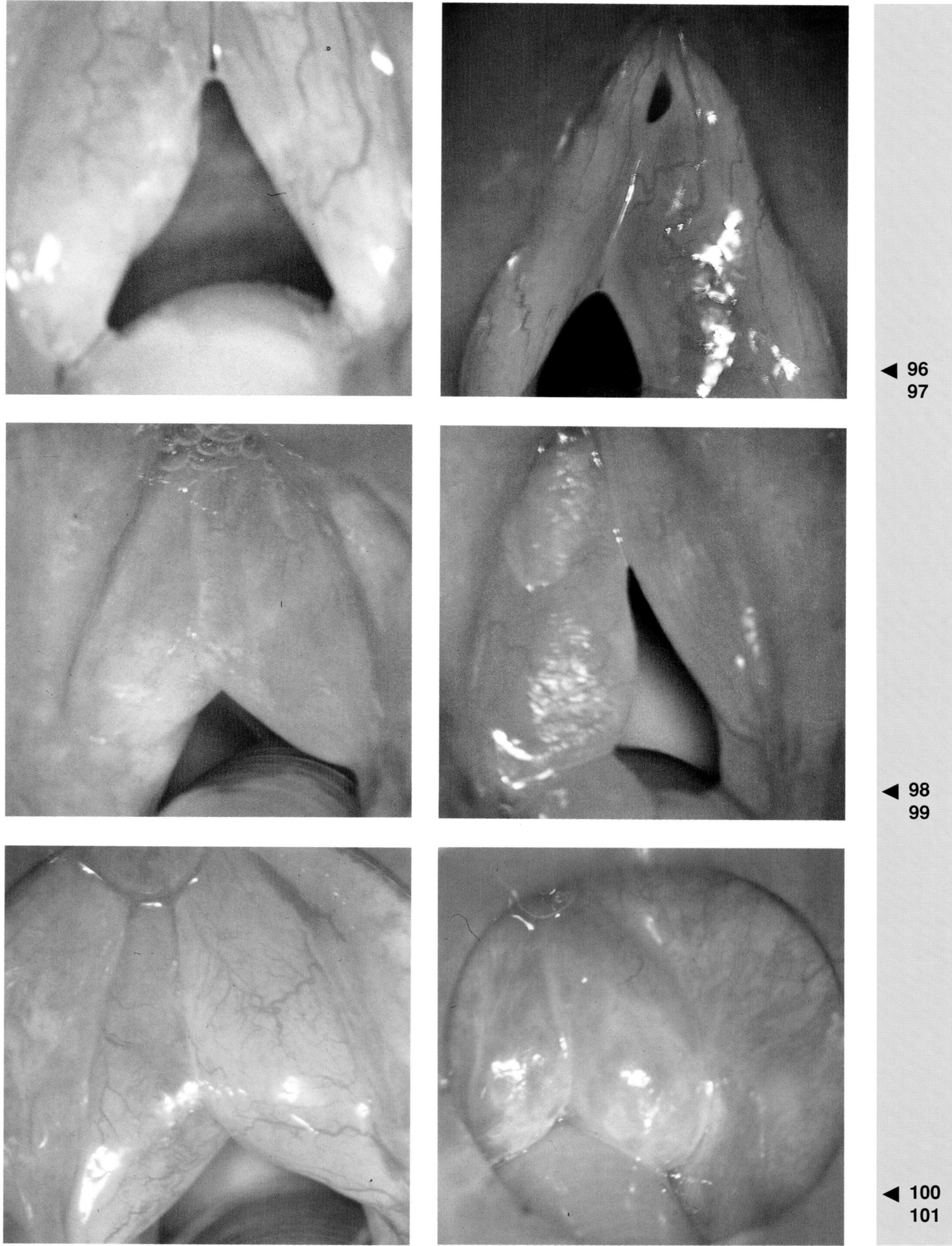

◀ 96
97

◀ 98
99

◀ 100
101

tion of synechia it is essential to preserve a few millimeters of mucosa on both sides at the anterior commissure, where in any case the edema is less pronounced. Removal of the edematous swelling with forceps alone almost always causes irregular mucosal edges that later form polypoid swellings leading to a very poor voice (Figure 102). The epithelial defect over the vocal cord should be as small as possible to shorten the period of re-epithelialization.[44] However, it is certainly an error to remove too little epithelium, because remnants of edema together with epithelial remnants produce an irregular surface on the vocal cord leading to poor functional results.

I have seen patients submitted elsewhere to the carbon dioxide laser in whom the edge of the vocal cord was tattooed by carbonized tissue at the point of impact of the laser beam.

Patients with very marked bilateral Reinke's edema are often aphonic for several weeks after the operation and often only learn to phonate again with the vocal cords with some difficulty. I remove most of the Reinke's edema in one sitting and have so far not produced webs at the anterior commissure. However, in well developed Reinke's edema with vestibular fold hyperplasia I now do the operation in two sittings 2 months apart to facilitate relearning of phonation. Postoperative speech therapy is often indicated in Reinke's edema.

A few cases of vestibular fold hyperplasia due to Reinke's edema require reduction in size of the vestibular fold by a wedge excision (page 75). Obviously the patient must stop smoking.

After removal of Reinke's edema, the mobile Reinke's space is lost and the epithelium lies directly on the vocal cord. Despite this, 90% of our patients claimed that they could produce a good voice and that their voice had improved considerably compared with its state before operation. In 5% of cases the voice was not improved, and in 5% it was worse.

I have never yet seen a recurrence of Reinke's edema after the technique described above, and indeed recurrence is not to be expected because the space is no longer present.

h. Chronic Hyperplastic Laryngitis (Figures 103–117)

Chronic hyperplastic laryngitis is uncommon in our series. However, only advanced cases come to microlaryngoscopy and many patients remain untreated.

More than 90% of the patients are men, most commonly in the fourth to sixth decades of life. The predilection for age and sex closely follows that for squamous cell carcinoma of the vocal cords, and furthermore 90% are cigarette smokers. Vocal abuse and the effect of gases, heat, and dust at work are said to be responsible for the development of chronic hyperplastic laryngitis, but they probably play a subordinate role in its pathogenesis.

Fig. 102.

This case of Reinke's edema has been treated by "stripping" of the vocal cords. A web has formed in the anterior commissure, and remnants of edematous tissue can be seen on both sides.

Fig. 103.

Early stage of chronic hyperplastic laryngitis: the epithelium is swollen and opaque due to hyperplasia at the anterior part of the vocal cords on both sides.

Fig. 104.

Chronic hyperplastic laryngitis in an early stage: bilateral epithelial hyperplasia is limited to the anterior segment of the vocal cords; the surface of the vocal cords shows early irregular contours.

Fig. 105.

Epithelial thickening due to chronic hyperplastic laryngitis extending from end-to-end of both vocal cords. The epithelium now resembles skin.

Fig. 106.

Chronic hyperplastic laryngitis which has now extended over both vocal cords. The irregular surface has undergone clear epidermization.

Fig. 107.

Chronic hyperplastic laryngitis: the epithelium is markedly thickened and keratinized, and the surface of the epithelium shows deposits of viscous and adherent mucus.

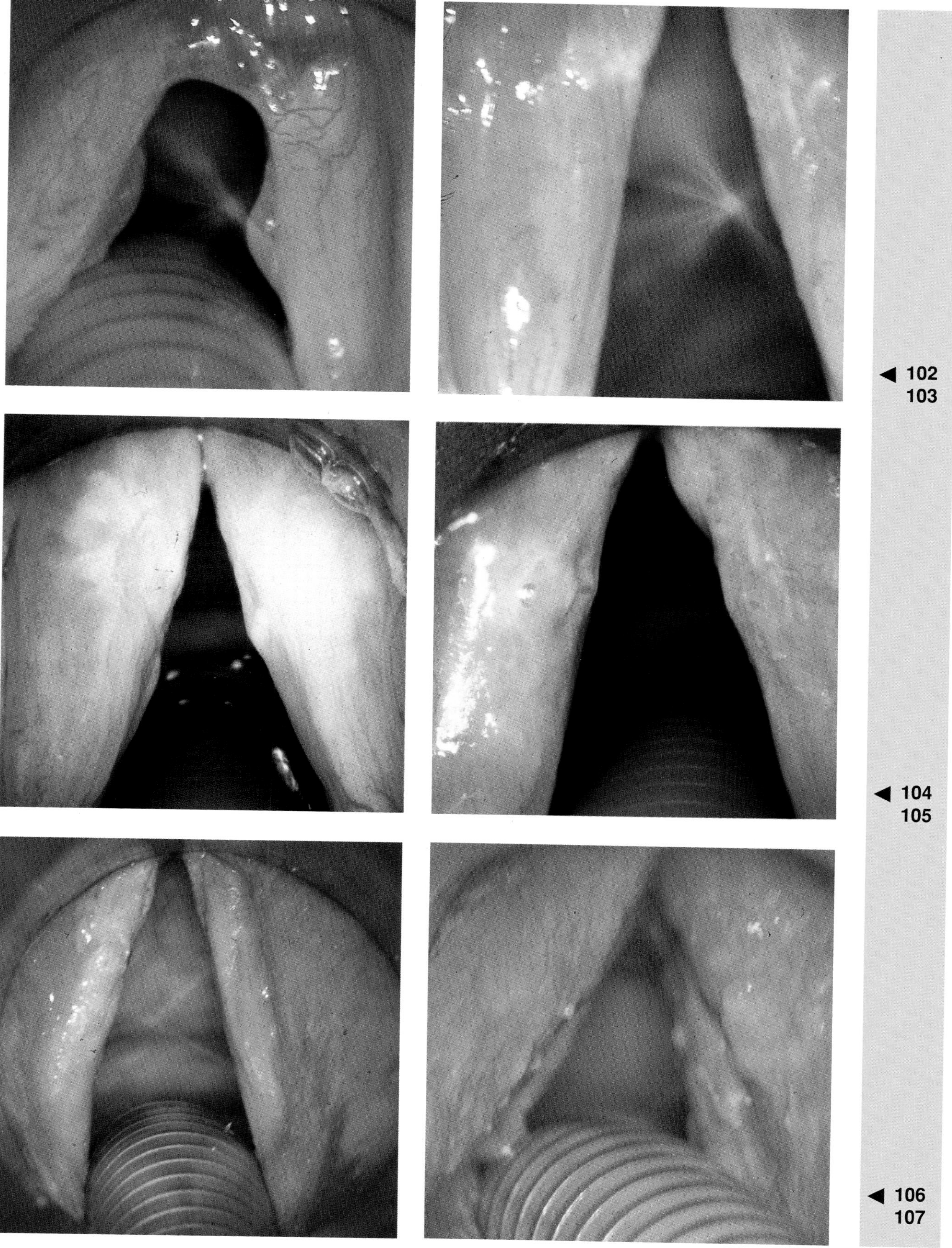

◀ 102
103

◀ 104
105

◀ 106
107

The disease always affects both vocal cords. The epithelium initially becomes thickened on the anterior part of the cords, and keratoses occur to some extent on the surface (Figures 103–104). The surface thus appears white, and the submucosal capillaries are concealed beneath this thickened layer. The previously thin, delicate squamous epithelium of the vocal cord gradually takes on the appearance of skin (Figure 105).

The process can be termed epidermization, an analogy to the similar lesion of the uterine cervix. In the early stages, the hyperplastic squamous epithelium is mobile over the vocal cords, but in more advanced stages Reinke's space is increasingly obliterated by inflammatory cell infiltrates and connective tissue (Figure 106). In the course of time the vocal cords develop a tumid, irregular outline and become obviously thicker. The hyperplasia of the squamous epithelium extends to the area surrounding the vocal cords, especially to the subglottic region where the squamous epithelium increasingly replaces the respiratory epithelium, so that the junction between the respiratory and squamous epithelium is displaced inferiorly. In advanced cases squamous cell metaplasia is also often found in the supraglottic space, initially in the form of islands that gradually merge. It is remarkable, however, that the ventricular epithelium is always spared. The epidermization is accompanied by dyschylic lesions; the secretion of the seromucinous glands becomes thickened, yellowish, and often tenacious (Figures 107, 108). Sometimes the secretion dries out and becomes crusted and difficult to expel. The progress of this primarily chronic inflammatory process is interrupted by acute exacerbations during which the vocal cords become crimson in color with occasional slit-like ulcers (Figures 109, 110). The epithelium of the floor of the ventricle may show marked inflammatory changes and protrude as red gelatinous edematous swellings. This appearance is incorrectly termed prolapse of the ventricle. The superficial keratinous layers are usually thin, patchy, or diffuse. Thick plaques resembling carcinoma are unusual (Figures 111, 112, 113).

Chronic hyperplastic laryngitis must be distinguished from keratoma, which is usually unilateral, well circumscribed, and not surrounded by metaplastic squamous epithelium. Verrucous acanthosis shows a very much better developed papillary surface with multiple projecting foci.

The differential diagnosis includes the ulcer seen in patients afflicted with severe and frequent coughing attacks in bronchitis or asthma. These cough-ulcers develop on both cords; they are covered by fibrin and mucus and are surrounded by thickened epithelium extending over the entire length of the membranous part of the vocal cords. The appearance strongly resembles that of the early stages of chronic hyperplastic laryngitis. In many patients the lesion resolves spontaneously if the coughing attacks cease, and the squamous epithelium of the vocal cords then regains its normal appearance. Microlaryngoscopy may be indicated in some cases for differential diagnosis, but operative treatment of this transient lesion is not indicated.

Histologic sections of the lesions of simple chronic hyperplastic laryngitis show a very thick squamous epithelium with pronounced acanthosis without nuclear atypia or disorders of stratification, but with parakeratosis of varying thickness. The submucous zone shows an inflammatory infiltrate of varying density and fibrosis of Reinke's space.

Fig. 108.

The entire surface of the larynx has become epidermized and is partially covered by tenacious mucus.

Fig. 109.

Chronic hyperplastic laryngitis in an acute exacerbation: the vocal cord epithelium is very reddened and swollen; a slit-like, fibrin-covered ulcer has developed in the center of the right vocal cord.

Fig. 110.

Chronic hyperplastic laryngitis: the left vocal cord shows a deep longitudinal furrow, probably due to previous inflammation and ulceration.

Fig. 111.

Chronic hyperplastic laryngitis with keratotic leukoplakia: this appearance cannot be distinguished with certainty from a carcinoma, not even by microlaryngoscopy. The thickened epithelium surrounding the keratin deposits demonstrates marked inflammation.

Fig. 112.

Chronic hyperplastic laryngitis with keratinization of the epithelium of the vocal cord and vestibular fold.

Fig. 113.

Same case as in Figure 112, after decortication of the vocal cord. The prolapsed ventricular epithelium and the leukoplakia of the right vestibular fold will be removed at a second sitting.

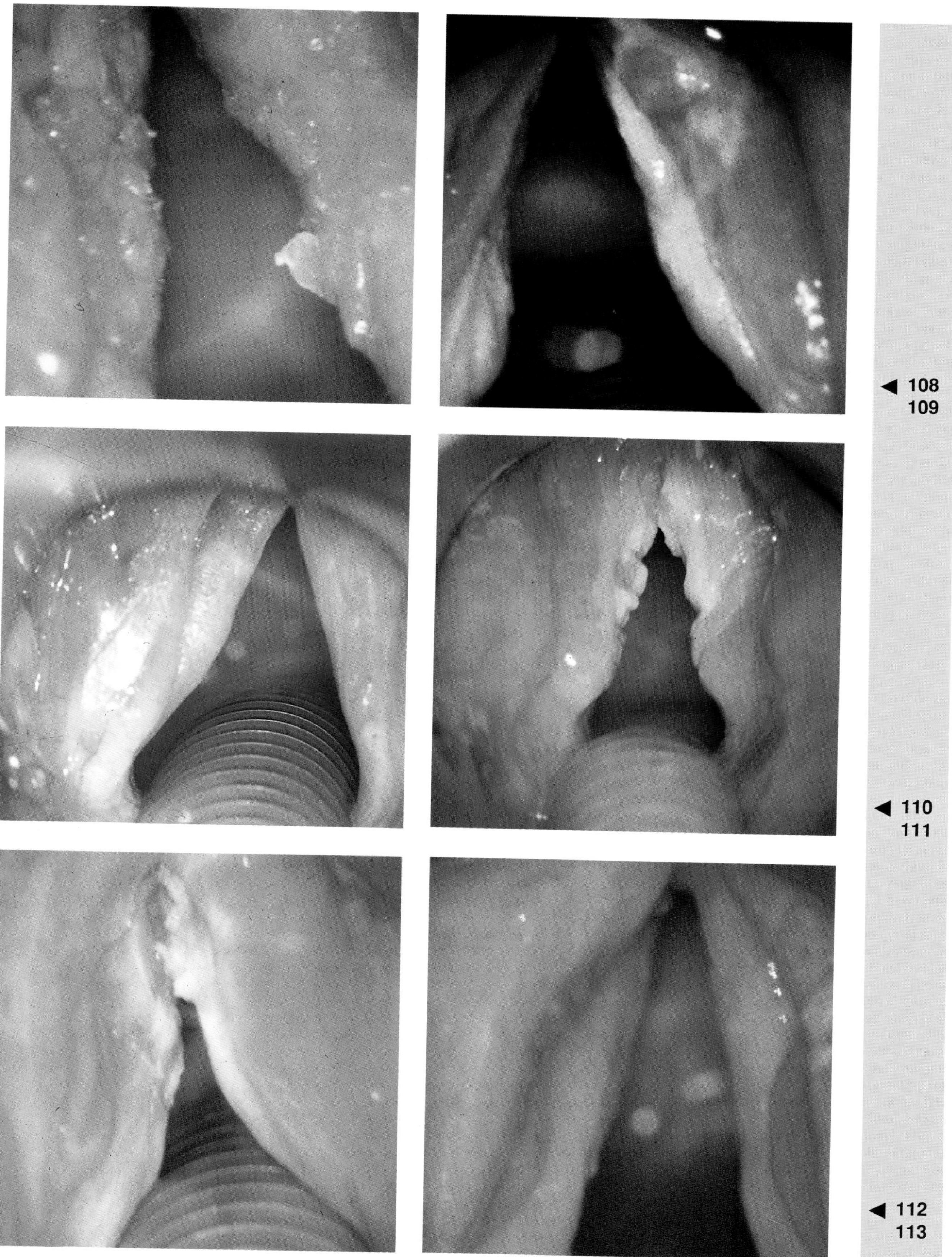

◀ 108
109

◀ 110
111

◀ 112
113

The **relation between chronic laryngitis and carcinoma is very important,**[7, 14] which is emphasized by the predilection for the same age, the same sex, and the fact that both diseases occur in cigarette smokers. About 6% of our patients with carcinoma of the vocal cords previously suffered chronic laryngitis, confirmed by biopsy, for at least 2 years before the appearance of the carcinoma.[14] Not every case of chronic laryngitis proceeds to carcinoma, nor does every carcinoma develop from chronic laryngitis, but chronic laryngitis must be regarded as a promoting factor.

The early stage of malignant degeneration (cancerization) of chronic hyperplastic laryngitis is very difficult to recognize by microlaryngoscopy (Figures 114–117). Individual projecting plaques, nodules, and ulcers must always be regarded with great suspicion. On several occasions I have been astonished when histologic examination of a specimen showed multiple malignant foci in the hyperplastic epithelium. In several of these cases the carcinoma arose directly from the basal layers in the absence of changes in the upper epithelial layers, hiding a malignant process lying more deeply.[14]

Treatment begins with inhalation therapy and strong advice to stop smoking, provided that there is no suspicion of carcinoma. Surgery should not be carried out during an acute exacerbation. However, the epithelial hyperplasia persists even after prolonged intensive convervative measures and after a certain stage is irreversible, so that almost all cases ultimately require surgery.

Surgery has three goals:

1. Removal of the hyperplastic epithelium to contribute to the healing of the inflammatory process.
2. Improvement of the voice by removal of the hyperplastic epithelium and submucous fibrosis. This requires remodeling of the vocal cord to resemble its natural state as closely as possible. The smooth surface of this remodeled vocal cord will allow better phonation.
3. Prophylaxis against the development of cancer and exclusion of an already established cancer.

   Surgery consists of very careful excision of the hyperplastic epithelium alone, if necessary in several sittings if the disease is widespread. The thickened epithelium should be stripped from the vocal ligament only in the very early stages. In more advanced cases I remove the epithelium in narrow strips, taking care not to damage the vocal ligament, which no longer presents a smooth layer. The operation is always carried out with sharp instruments, with the most careful preservation of the vocal ligament, and not by stripping. The operation is followed by intensive treatment with inhalations. Voice conservation and the avoidance of cigarette smoking should be continued, and speech therapy should begin **after** the operation.

Fig. 114.

Chronic hyperplastic laryngitis that has undergone malignant degeneration: the typical inflammatory changes can still be recognized on the right vocal cord, whereas on the left side there is a partially ulcerated squamous carcinoma extending into the vestibular fold.

Fig. 115.

Chronic laryngitis that has undergone malignant degeneration. This patient had been under follow-up for 10 years for chronic hyperplastic laryngitis and now shows multicentric carcinoma on both vocal cords.

Fig. 116.

Category T3 carcinoma of the right vocal cord of a patient with chronic hyperplastic laryngitis. On the left side the entire vocal cord has undergone epidermization.

Fig. 117.

Multicentric malignant change on both right and left sides in chronic hyperplastic laryngitis.

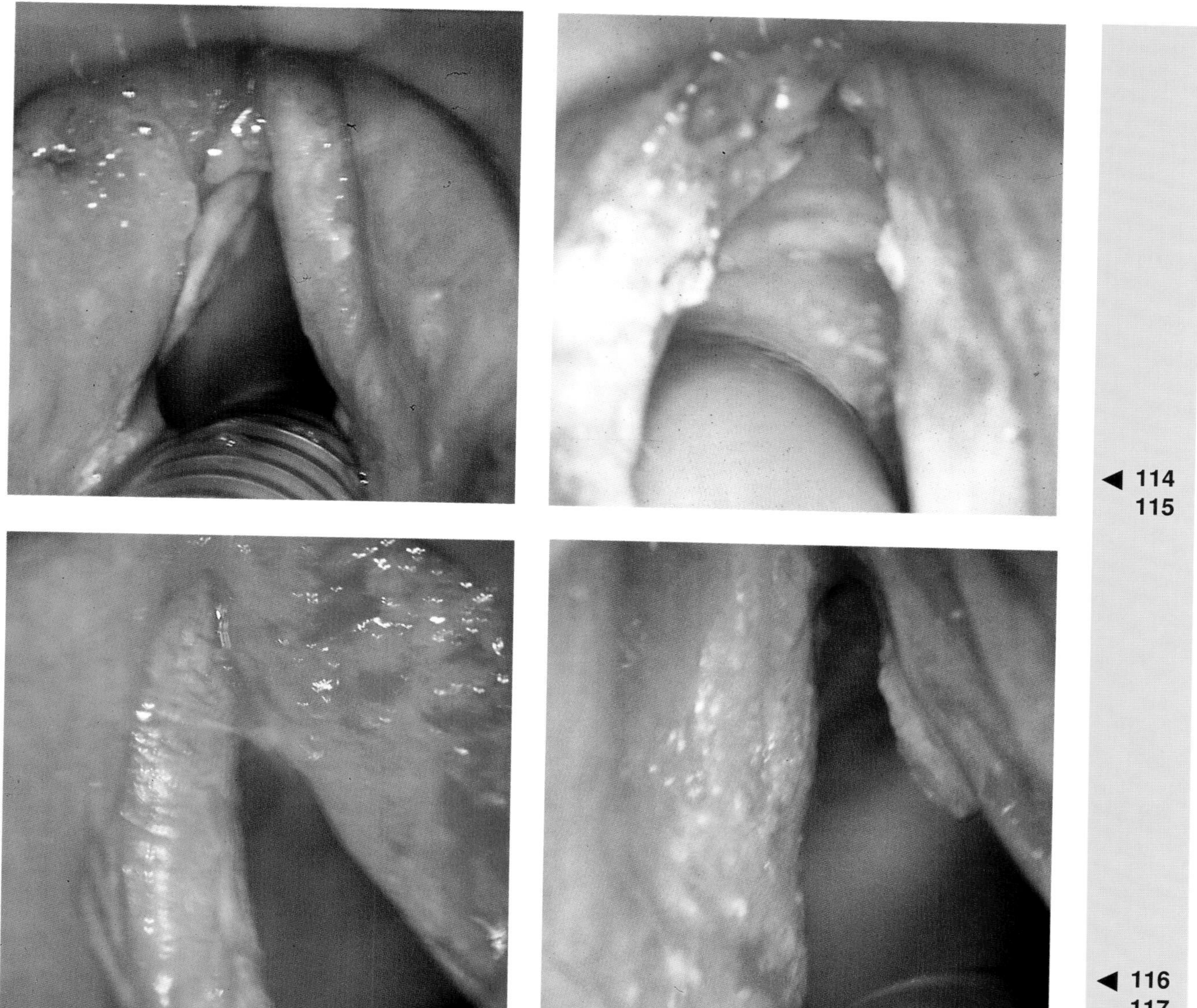

◀ 114
115

◀ 116
117

i. Interarytenoid Pachydermia (Figures 118–119)

This unusual lesion affects adults of both sexes equally. It is characterized by mounds of thickened epithelium lying between the arytenoid cartilages. The thickened epithelium is wrinkled and sometimes projects like a cockscomb into the glottis during phonation. A few cases also show mucous deposits and fine keratinization of the surface (Figures 118, 119). Interarytenoid pachydermia does not need to be removed because carcinoma almost never arises in this area; furthermore, removal of the tissue could well be followed by scar formation of the posterior part of the larynx, leading to limitation of vocal cord mobility.

j. Specific Forms of Laryngitis

1. Tuberculosis (Figures 120–123)

Laryngeal tuberculosis was very familiar to earlier generations of laryngologists but has now become so unusual that the disease is often forgotten and remains undiagnosed unless proven pulmonary tuberculosis provides a clue.

In a new case of mucosal tuberculosis the multiple small red miliary tubercles can be recognized lying just beneath the mucosa. In a few cases the tubercles may become confluent to form polypoid nodules that can caseate (Figures 120–122) and form small ulcers. Large tuberculomas especially affect the supraglottic part or the posterior wall of the larynx (Figure 123). Tuberculous granulomas are usually surrounded by highly inflamed reddened mucosa. Laryngeal tuberculosis is most often confused with carcinoma, polyps, or chronic laryngitis. The treatment is entirely by chemotherapy once the diagnosis has been made by biopsy or culture. I have not observed the laryngeal stenosis that so often followed the healing of laryngeal tuberculosis in earlier times.

Fig. 118.
Interarytenoid pachydermia with flat, leathery epithelial thickening of the posterior wall of the larynx.

Fig. 119.
Interarytenoid pachydermia with fine papillary wrinkled epithelium of the posterior wall of the larynx.

Fig. 120.
Tuberculosis of the right vocal cord with several submucosal tubercles and collateral subglottic crimson edema.

Fig. 121.
Vocal cord tuberculosis showing individual tubercles on both vocal cords.

Fig. 122.
Tuberculous ulcer on the laryngeal surface of the epiglottis.

Fig. 123.
Necrotizing tuberculosis on the left side of the epiglottis.

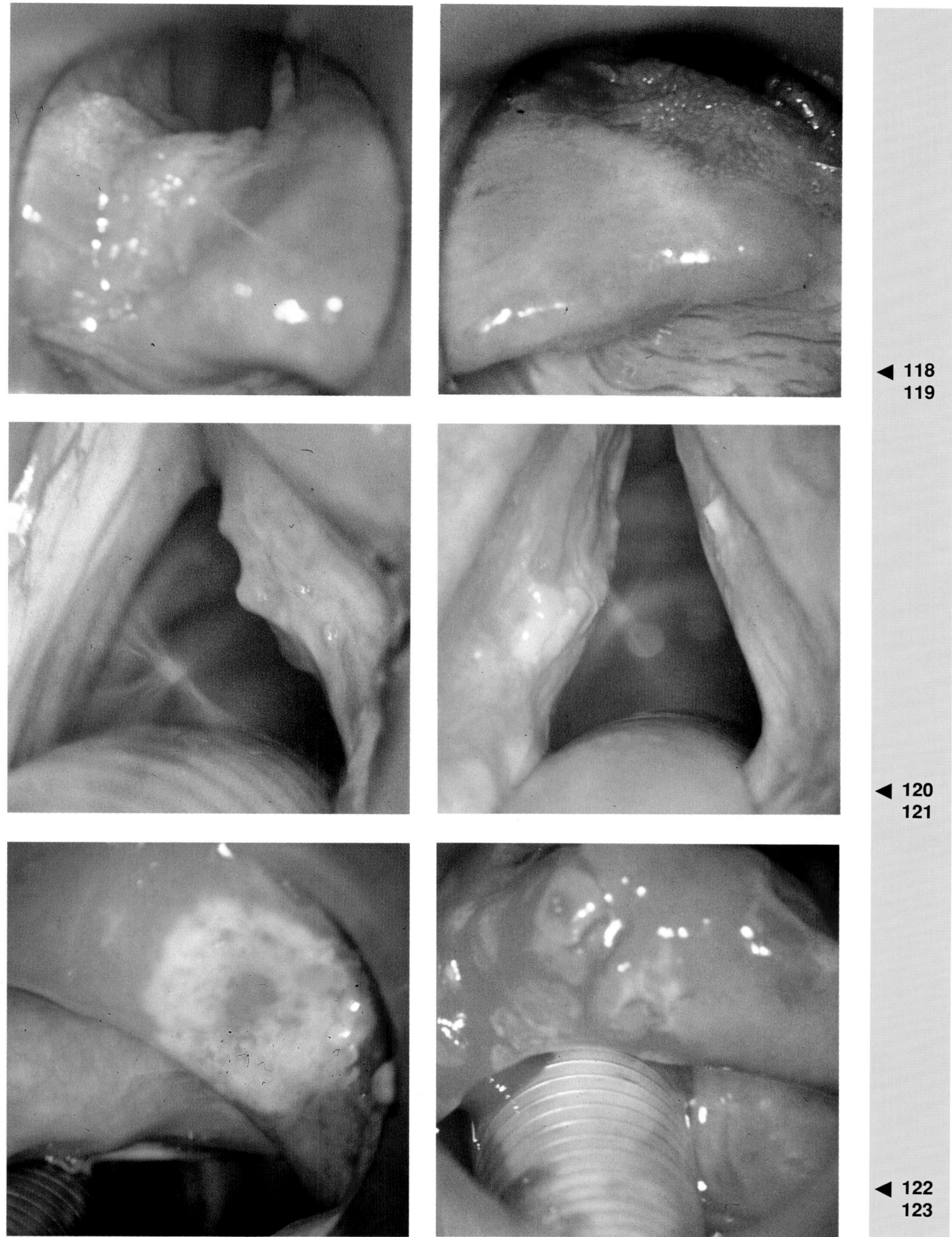

◀ 118
119

◀ 120
121

◀ 122
123

2. Sarcoidosis (Figures 124–128)

In recent years I have seen several examples of laryngeal sarcoidosis, mainly in young men. A highly characteristic diffuse swelling of the epiglottis and the aryepiglottic folds is the most common finding (Figures 124, 125, 126). Palpation shows the swelling to be firm, rubbery, and usually limited to the supraglottic space. The patient complains neither of pain nor of other symptoms, and tracheotomy is seldom needed. Two of our cases showed sarcoidosis affecting the vestibular fold and the vocal cord (Figures 127, 128). The extensive thickenings with a slightly papillary surface were firm in consistency.[53]

The diagnosis is confirmed by histological demonstration of noncaseating epitheloid cell granulomas. It is sometimes difficult to take a biopsy that incorporates a typical granuloma. In our cases the laryngeal sarcoidosis was the only manifestation of the disease.

Surgery is not indicated. The swelling can usually be reduced in size by steroids, but cessation of treatment is followed by rapid recurrence, so that prolonged treatment is essential. The course of the disease is difficult to predict; several of our patients have been suffering from this disease for several years.

3. Syphilis (Figure 129)

A new case of laryngeal syphilis is now an exceedingly rare occurrence, although defects, scars, and stenosis occasionally seen due to a healed syphilitic granuloma are seen.

4. Scleroma

Scleroma of the larynx has become so unusual in central Europe that not one single case has been seen in the Marburg Clinic in the last 15 years. However, scleroma is still seen relatively often in Central and South America and in Egypt.[57]

5. Mycoses

Infection of the larynx by **candida albicans** leads to the development of tumor-like white viscous infiltrates and fixation of the vocal cords. The infection may also spread to the laryngeal skeleton, to be followed by laryngeal stenosis.

Fig. 124.

Diffuse thickening of the epiglottis and both aryepiglottic folds in laryngeal sarcoid.

Fig. 125.

Laryngeal sarcoid in which the epiglottis has become tubular as a result of inflammatory granulation.

Fig. 126.

Laryngeal sarcoid. In this case the epiglottis and the aryepiglottic fold were so thickened that the patient required a temporary tracheostomy.

Fig. 127.

Sarcoidosis of the left vestibular fold and the left vocal cord showing extensive diffuse swelling, of firm consistency.

Fig. 128.

Sarcoidosis of both vestibular folds and vocal cords causing marked narrowing of the laryngeal lumen.

Fig. 129.

Long-standing syphilitic scars on the epiglottis.

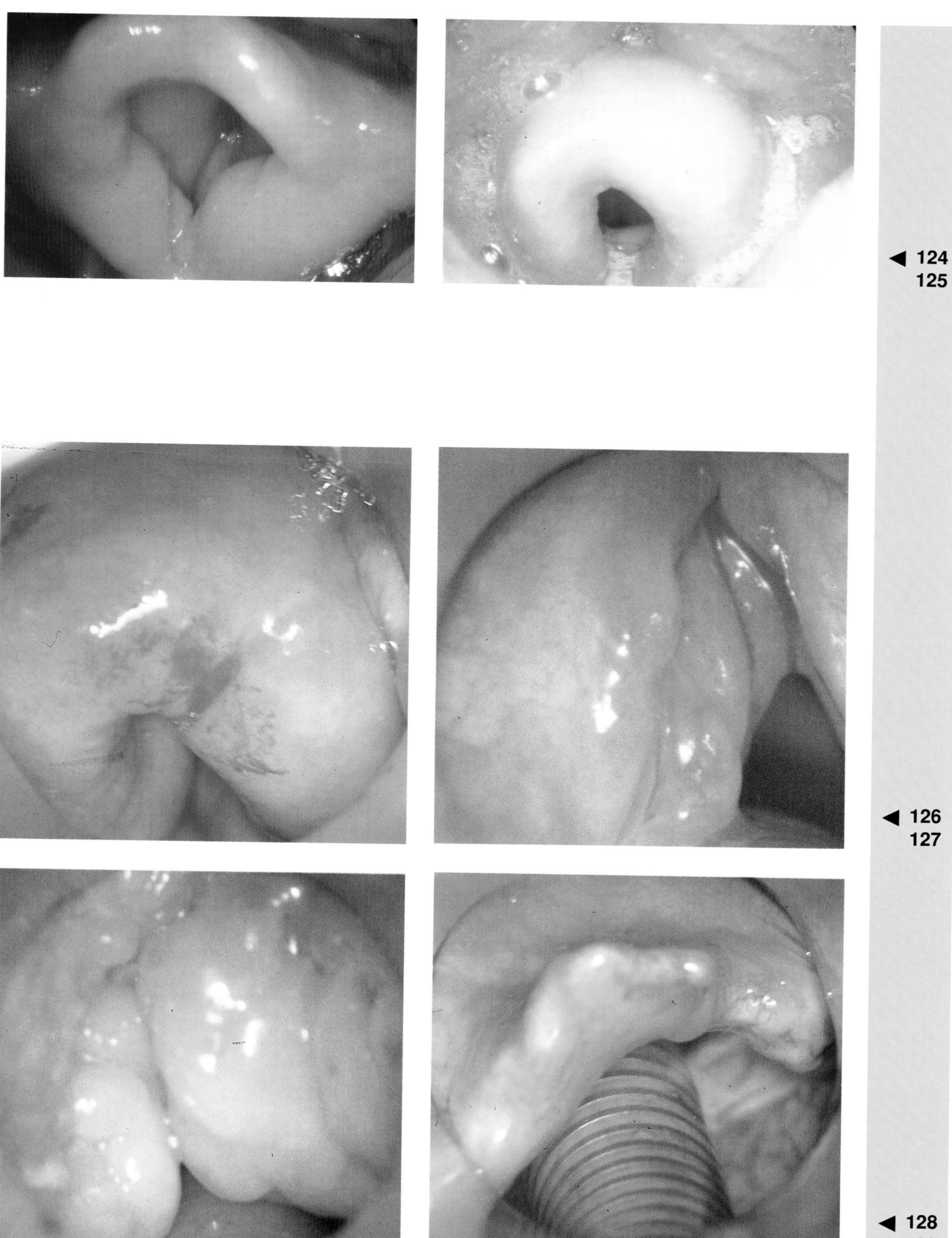

◀ 124
125

◀ 126
127

◀ 128
129

k. Juvenile Papillomatosis (Figures 130–139)

Juvenile papillomas are probably caused by a virus, although so far this virus has neither been identified by immunology nor electromicroscopy. Males are much more often affected than females.

Age distribution shows a clear peak between the ages of 4 and 6 and a further one between the third and fifth decades of life. The disease is characterized by recurrent **multiple** papillomas, whereas adult (senile) papillomas are always single with keratinization of the surface (page 99).

Juvenile papillomas always begin on the vocal cords and then often extend to the supra – and infraglottic areas (Figures 130, 131). In extreme cases the papillomas may extend either as a continuous sheet or as discrete lesions over the entire pharynx as far as the roof of the nasopharynx, or inferiorly into the trachea and bronchi, a much more dangerous event.

Small papillomas form smooth, finely granular red sheets that may project only a little above the level of the surrounding laryngeal mucosa (Figures 132, 133) but are usually more papilliferous and sometimes even form cauliflower-like pedicled masses (Figures 134–139). High magnification shows small apical capillaries on the surface of the individual villi. Keratinization is unusual and sparse.

The branching villi of a papilloma are covered by a multilayered cuboidal epithelium, often with impressive large round dark nuclei but seldom with coarser nuclear atypia. Many papillomas, particularly those that recur rapidly, may be highly cellular and appear premalignant to the relatively inexperienced pathologist. Mitoses are occasionally seen but nuclear dysplasia is absent.

Numerous methods such as ultrasound, cryoprobes, various chemotherapeutic agents, interferon, and so forth have been tried for the treatment of juvenile papillomas but then abandoned.[58] All of these methods, even if they have any effect at all, are purely symptomatic since the disease has an immunobiological basis that we are so far incapable of modifying. The possibility and frequency of recurrence are determined not by the skills of the laryngologist and the methods at his disposal, but by immunological events. In the absence of any treatment for the basic cause, the main principles of management are thorough removal of the papillomas, avoiding the production of scar tissue, restoring the voice, and maintaining an airway. Simple removal of the papillomas using a cupped forceps usually leads to brisk hemorrhage, so that the method usually recommended is vaporization of the papillomas by the laser.[6]

In my experience removal with the suction coagulator is simpler, quicker, and neater. The microcoagulator probe is applied to the papillomas and the high frequency current set low enough to ensure that the papillomas are not charred but are converted into a fluid that can be sucked off easily. Even the most extensive papillomas can be removed quickly in this way without damage to the underlying tissue. Existing scars and webs should be removed endoscopically together with the papillomas.

Fig. 130.
Small juvenile papilloma of the right vocal cord.

Fig. 131.
Juvenile nonkeratinizing papilloma of the right vocal cord.

Fig. 132.
Bilateral papilloma sheets extending over both vocal cords.

Fig. 133.
Papillomas occupying the right vocal cord at the anterior commissure. This case demonstrates the relatively nonprojecting, field-like form of juvenile papillomatosis.

Fig. 134.
Papillomatosis of the entire glottis in an infant showing the more pendulous form of papilloma.

Fig. 135.
Juvenile papillomas at the anterior commissure and the subglottis.

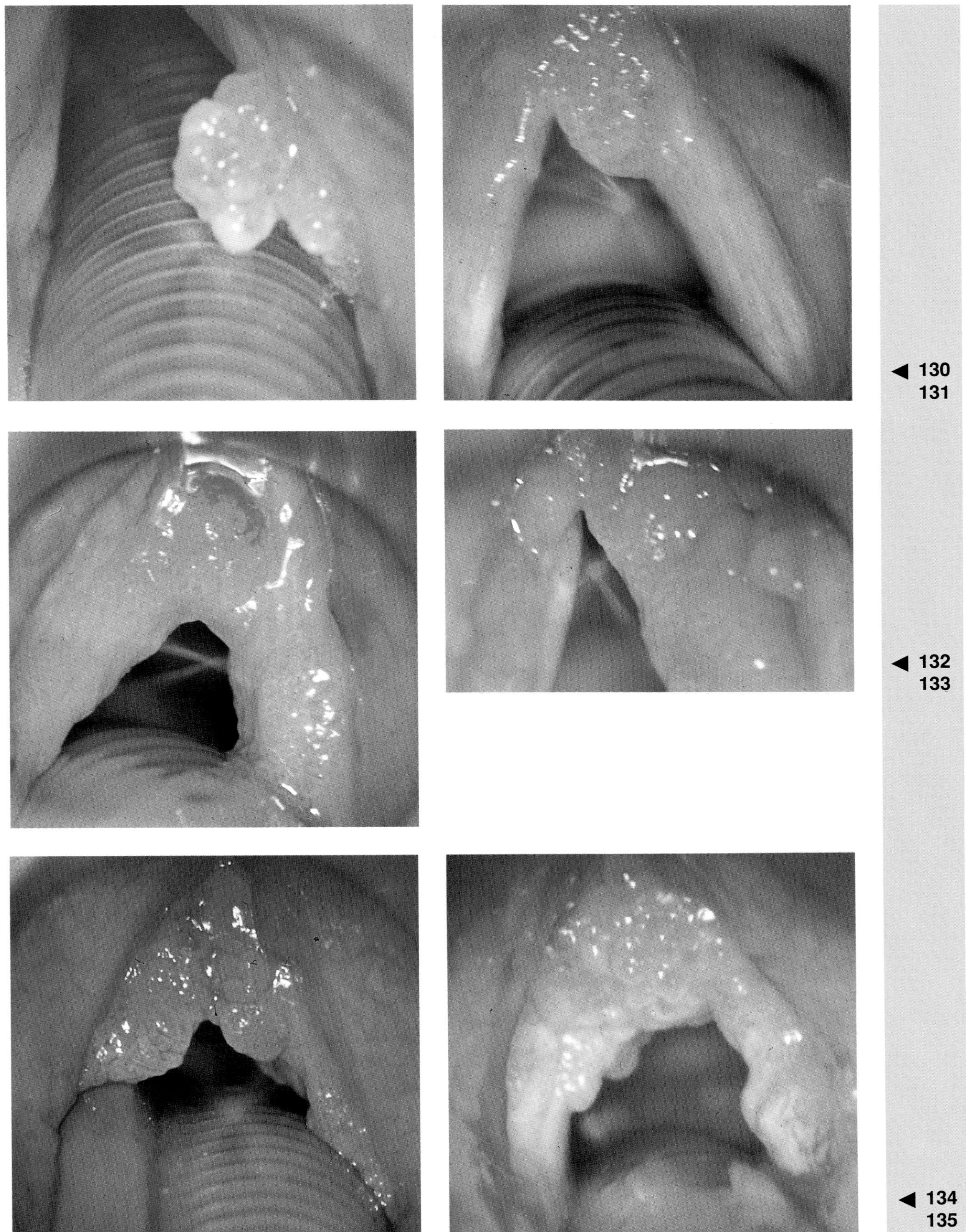

◀ 130
131

◀ 132
133

◀ 134
135

The most recent advances thus consist not of treatment of the cause of the papillomas but of exact surgery and the prevention of the scars that so often follow the removal of these lesions. It is now possible to avoid a tracheotomy, which previously was so often necessary. It is completely impossible to forecast the course of papillomatosis in the individual case. As a rule of thumb it can be said that papillomas in young children grow and recur particularly quickly, whereas the course of the disease in older children and adults is slower. Typically juvenile papillomas recur not only at the site from which they have previously been removed but in ever wider areas of the laryngeal mucosa. Some cases undergo spontaneous resolution for no obvious reason and then recur again many years later. Some patients never achieve healing, even over a period of decades, but suffer repeated recurrences. Puberty has no obvious influence on the resolution of papillomatosis.

Only in very rare cases does adult laryngeal or bronchial carcinoma arise from papillomatosis. Most of such patients have previously been smokers. The frequency of carcinoma arising from juvenile papillomatosis is so small that it can be ignored in practice.[30] There are earlier descriptions of cases in which irradation of the papillomas was followed by radiation-induced carcinoma.

I. Single Papilloma (Figure 140)

Small nonkeratinized pharyngeal papillomas arising from the uvula in the anterior palatine arch are familiar to every ENT surgeon. These are usually completely innocent, coincidental findings.

Similar papillomas affecting the aryepiglottic fold, the arytenoid, or the epiglottis are rarely found.

Fig. 136.
Juvenile papilloma of the left vestibular fold.

Fig. 137.
Extensive papillomatosis of the entire larynx.

Fig. 138.
The same case as in Figure 137 showing the epiglottis covered by a sheet of papilloma.

Fig. 139.
A pendulous cluster of papilloma obstructing the laryngeal inlet.

Fig. 140.
a) A pedicled papilloma hanging from the epiglottis and resembling uvular papilloma. b) Surgical specimen.

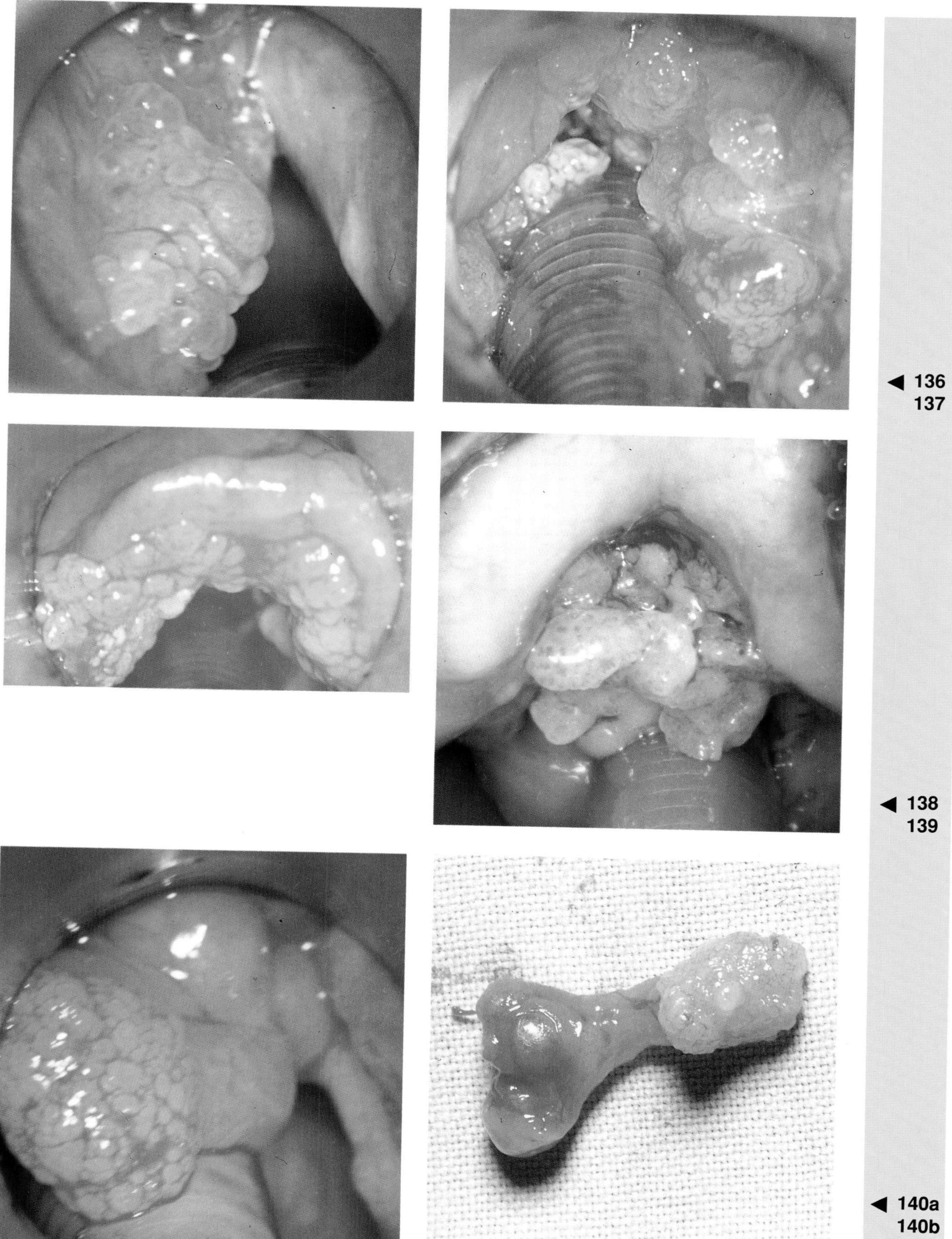

◀ 136
137

◀ 138
139

◀ 140a
140b

m. Verrucous Acanthosis (Verrucous Carcinoma) (Figures 141–147)

This relatively rare disease is classified by most authors as a subgroup of squamous call carcinomas. However, metastases or histologically confirmed infiltration has not been demonstrated in any of the cases described so far. Furthermore, in a personal series followed up for 10 years or more, no patient has developed metastases, and we therefore believe that this lesion is not a carcinoma but probably a viral disease.[15]

Verrucous acanthosis is characterized by the development of extensive proliferations covered by thick layers of keratin. These proliferations may spread over the vocal cord, vestibular fold, and epiglottis (Figures 141–143). Multiple satellite foci are relatively frequent (Figure 141). The wart-like white plaques or bark-like structures extend widely, adhere firmly to the underlying tissue, and are difficult to remove (Figure 144). They look like tumors but remain always superficial and do not infiltrate the underlying tissue.

Histologic examination of as much material as possible is required to establish the diagnosis with certainty and to differentiate the lesion from a highly differentiated squamous cell carcinoma with verrucous morphology. Microscopy shows ribbons of enfolded and warty keratinized epithelial masses projecting as thick plump pegs that always have a sharp boundary. Crypts like those in the tonsil often contain plugs of debris, and keratin granulomas are also quite common. The plump acanthotic pegs are often surrounded by a marked inflammatory infiltrate consisting mainly of lymphocytes and leukocytes.

In recent years I have treated all cases by endoscopy. The leathery white plaques are dissected out using sharp instruments such as small scissors or a knife.

In many cases I have also used suction coagulation to allow piecemeal removal of the thickened diseased mucosa. Several sittings are advisable for extensive verrucous acanthosis. Recurrences (Figure 145–147) are fairly common, demanding repeat surgery, but I have not yet seen a single case of malignant degeneration.

Fig. 141.

Multiple foci of verrucous acanthosis extending over both vocal cords, with subglottic tumor on the right side also seen.

Fig. 142.

Verrucous acanthosis extending over the epiglottis.

Fig. 143.

Verrucous acanthosis showing thick plaques of epithelium on the left vestibular fold extending down to the vocal cord.

Fig. 144.

Recurrent tumor in the patient shown in Figure 143. Bark-like epithelial thickening of the left vocal cord.

Fig. 145.

Recurrent verrucous acanthosis. Thickened epithelium is again forming on the left vocal cord one year after decortication.

Fig. 146.

Verrucous acanthosis of both vocal cords.

Fig. 147.

Same case as in Figure 146 showing a rapidly progressing lesion on the left vocal cord 3 months after removal of the lesion on the right side. This patient remained free of recurrence for 2 years after removal of this lesion.

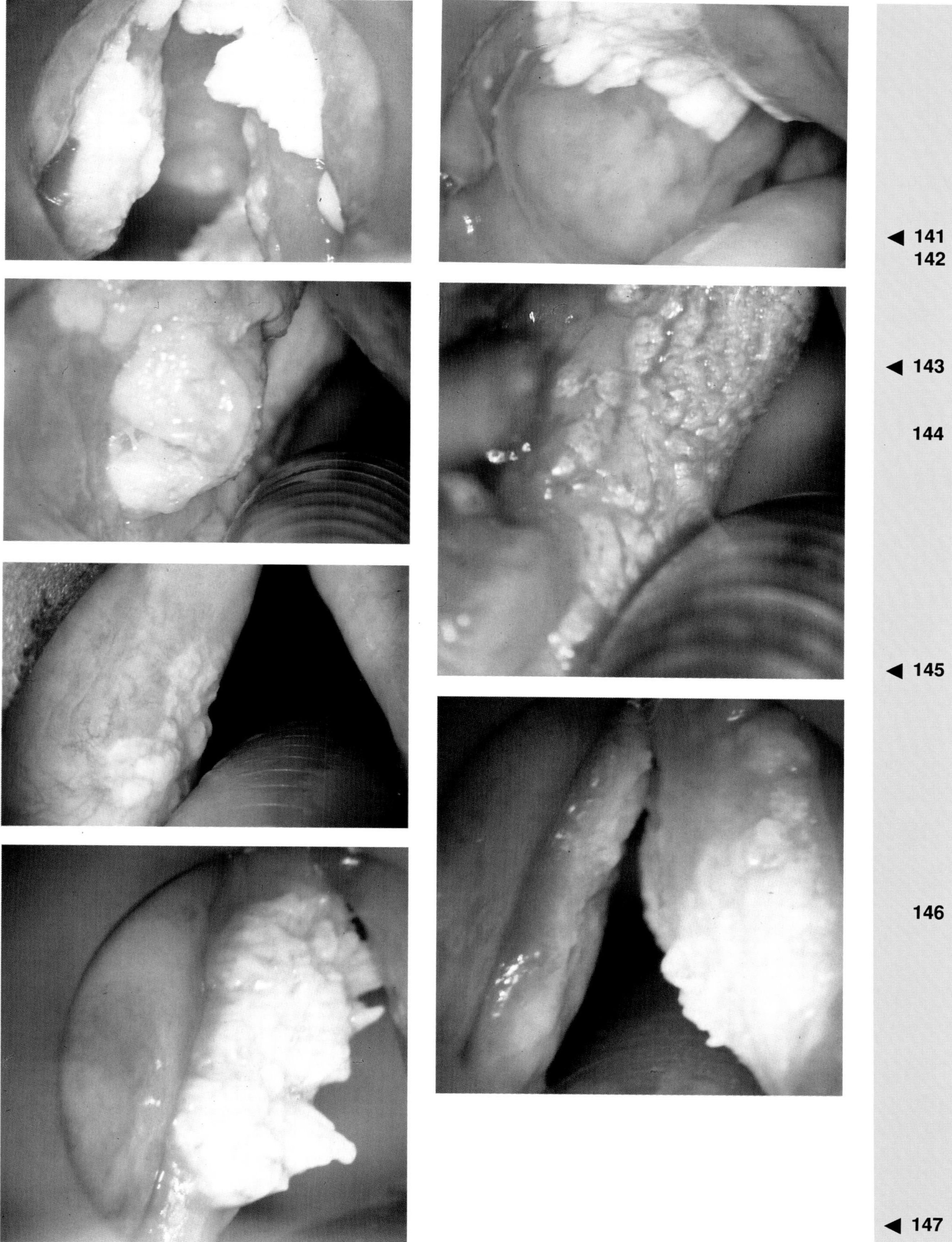

◀ 141
142
◀ 143
144
◀ 145
146
◀ 147

n. Amyloid Deposits (Figure 148–151)

Amyloid deposits in the larynx are not uncommon. They affect men and women with the same frequency, usually in the middle years of life.[46]

Small isolated amyloid deposits on the vocal cords resemble cysts or polyps (Figure 148). However, most amyloid deposits lie in the vestibular folds and form an "amyloid tumor" (Figures 149, 150). A few cases show extensive multiple deposits (Figure 151). Microlaryngoscopy shows a diffuse or more nodular swelling on one or both vocal cords or the vestibular fold and sometimes an extensive tumorlike appearance. The mucosa over the amyloid deposit is smooth and relatively avascular. Incision of the mucosa immediately reveals the characteristic avascular, yellowish, and friable amyloid deposit, which is often in clumps. Amyloidosis is identified histologically by the round hyaline deposits that stain with Congo red and can be identified by polarized light and by the foreign body giant cells surrounding the deposit.

An attempt is made to remove the individual clumps of amyloid piecemeal from the depth of the tissue. Unfortunately, they often infiltrate the vocal cord musculature or the vestibular fold completely. The technique should be as atraumatic as possible to preserve laryngeal function. It is usually impossible and unnecessary to remove extensive amyloid deposits completely, and it is then preferable to leave behind some clumps of the amyloid in order to preserve reasonable laryngeal function. External operation via a laryngofissure as formerly done is not indicated. In many cases the process is stationary, so that recurrence may be delayed for many years. However, other patients are afflicted by rapid progress with recurrent and enlarging amyloid deposits demanding repeated surgery.

Fig. 148.

Small bilateral emploid deposits within the vocal cords covered by thin edematous mucosa.

Fig. 149.

Amyloid tumor of the left vestibular fold. The vocal cord is completely obscured by a diffuse swelling of the vestibular fold that is hard on palpation.

Fig. 150.

Same case as in Figure 149, 6 months after excision of the lesion from the vestibular fold. A further amyloid deposit has now apperared on the right vestibular fold.

Fig. 151.

Extensive amyloid deposits in the entire supraglottic region of the larynx.

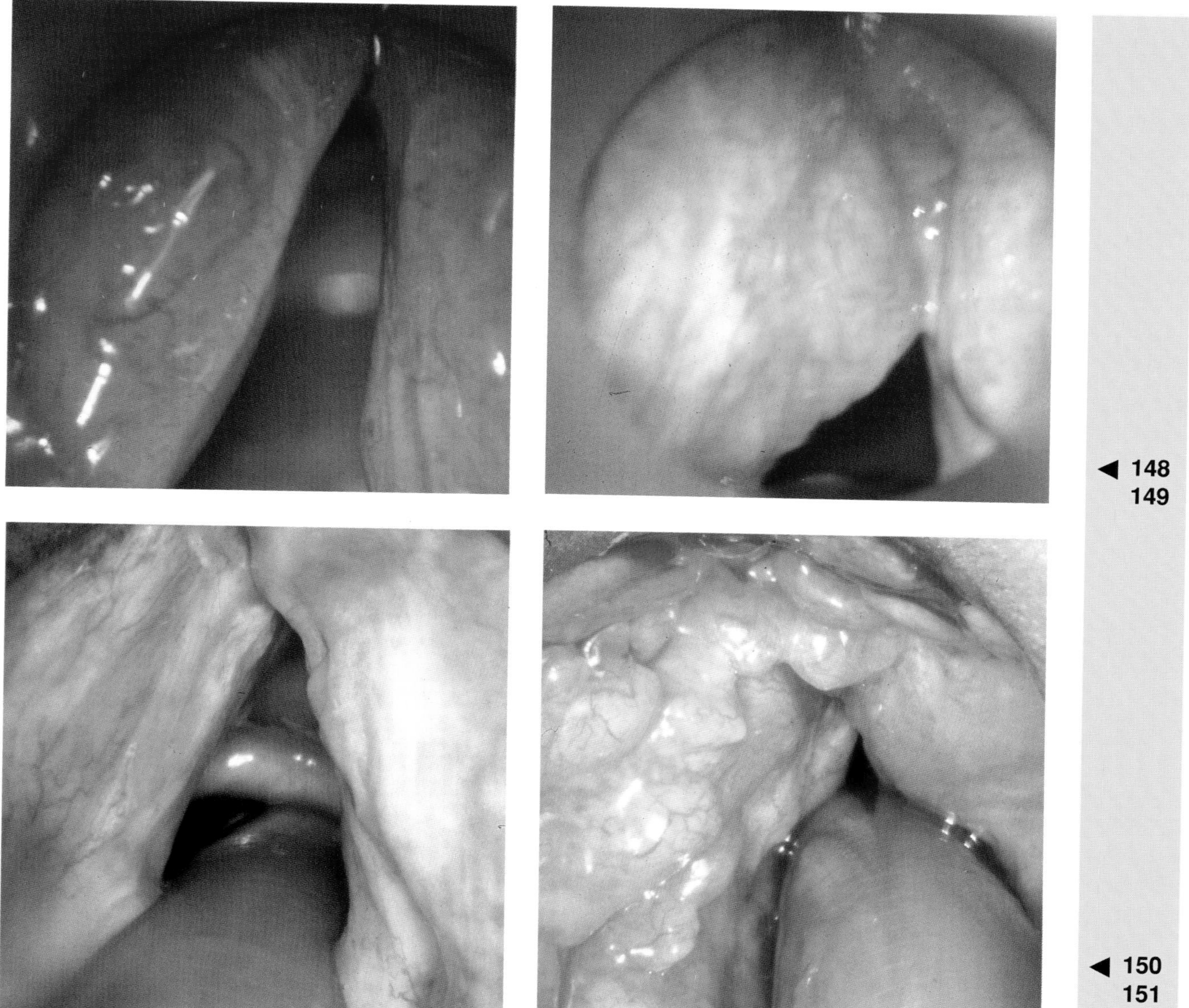

◀ 148
149

◀ 150
151

o. Hyperplasia of the Vestibular Fold (Figures 152–155)

Thickening of the vestibular fold has many causes,[34] the commonest being a cyst, and more rarely spastic dysphonia or vicarious hyperplasia in patients who are no longer able to phonate with the vocal cords because of paralysis, Reinke's edema, tumor, or defects.

These secondary forms of vestibular fold hyperplasia begin in the anterior part of the fold and extend gradually over the middle and posterior segments (Figures 152, 153, 154). A sphincter capable of active and independent motion develops, even if both vocal cords are paralyzed. This effect is a clear proof of motor fibers running in the superior laryngeal nerve. Material removed from such thickened vestibular folds, particularly in spastic dysphonia, often demonstrates striated muscle fibers that can only have arisen from the ventricularis muscle.

Supraglottic phonation (dysphonia plica ventricularis) can be produced by closing movements of the supraglottic sphincter. In many cases this may be highly desirable, for example if phonation with the glottis is no longer possible after resection or paralysis of the vocal cord.

In spastic dysphonia (in my view a result of dysfunction of the coordination between the glottic and supraglottic sphincters), the hypertrophic vestibular fold can be submitted to wedge resection to impede closure of the supraglottic sphincter. However, this long established procedure gives indifferent results. Excision of tissue from the vestibular folds is simple: the mucosa in the anterior two-thirds is incised in a half-moon shape, large pieces of tissue are removed from within the vestibular fold, the wound bed is coagulated, and finally the wound is closed with a few sutures (Figure 155).

Fig. 152.

Secondary vestibular fold hyperplasia in an early stage in a patient with hyperkinetic dysphonia. Only the anterior parts of the vestibular folds are thickened.

Fig. 153.

Secondary vestibular fold hyperplasia with coexistent atrophy of the vocal cords.

Fig. 154.

Secondary vicarious vestibular fold hyperplasia in Reinke's edema.

Fig. 155.

Surgical reduction of the vestibular fold. A half-moon-shaped segment is excised from the mucosa of the vestibular fold and from the quadrangular membrane. The underlying fat and the glandular tissue are then removed until the normal shape of the vestibular fold is restored.

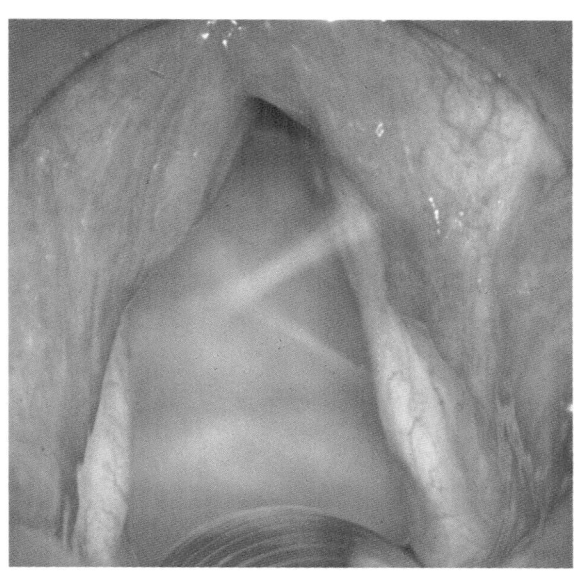

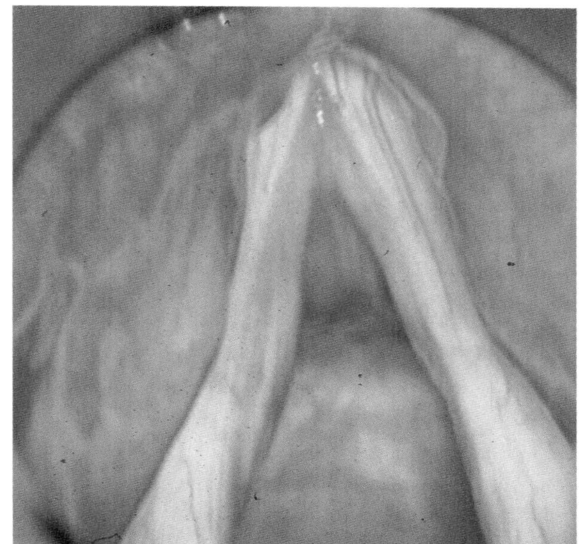

◀ 152
153

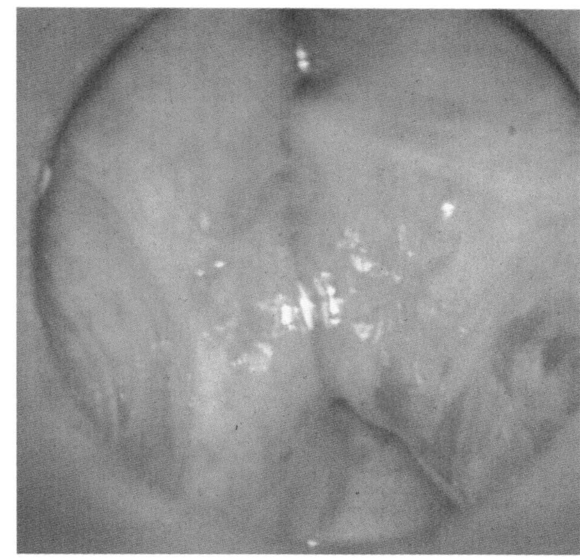

◀ 154

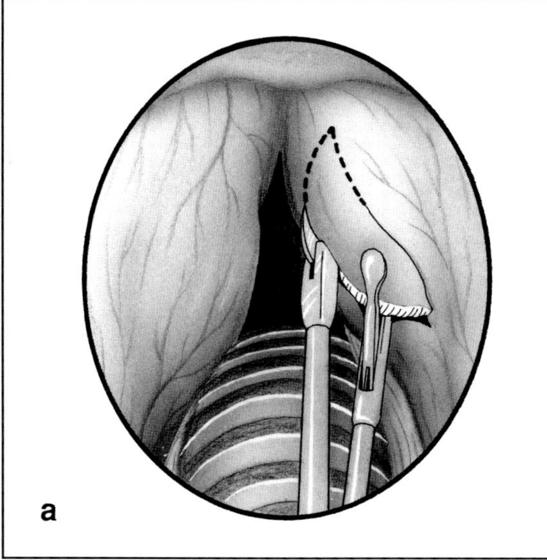

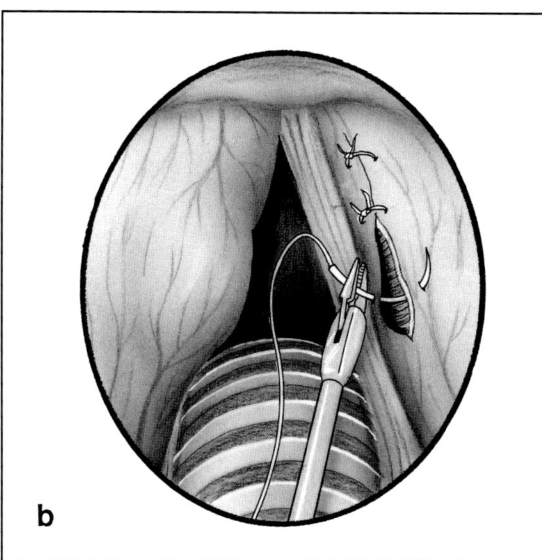

◀ 155

3. Trauma

a. Laryngeal Injury Due to Intubation

Intubation anesthesia or respiratory therapy can cause various lesions of the larynx that require surgery. The cause of these lesions is abrasion of the larynx by the endotracheal tube or the inflatable cuff, particularly if the anesthesia is too light and allows the patient to cough, retch, or move. The poor general condition of a patient subjected to artificial respiration over a prolonged period encourages the development of ulceration. Even high-volume low-pressure cuffs can produce abrasions extending as far as the esophagus. Regurgitation of gastric acid collecting above the cuff can cause serious mucosal lesions. Finally, the cause of the injury may be an endotracheal tube that is too large. Eighty percent of all intubation granulomas arise in women, which is certain evidence that the endotracheal tube is often too large for the small female larynx.

1. Fibrinous Ulcerative Laryngitis (Figures 156, 157)

Laryngoscopy carried out after endotracheal anesthesia almost always reveals inflammation of the vocal cords and sometimes a circumscribed fibrin membrane, particularly over the arytenoid cartilages; these lesions usually heal spontaneously.

However, in a few cases severe fibrinous ulcerative laryngitis can develop after even a brief intubation, possibly due to an allergic reaction to the material used in the manufacture of the tube or to regurgitated gastric acid. I have seen two cases of marked stridor after intubation with rubber tubes due to diffuse swelling of the vocal cords, which were covered extensively by fibrin. The swelling also extended into the subglottic region (Figures 156, 157). These cases resolved with repeated endoscopic suction and removal of the fibrin membrane, antibiotics, and decongestants.

2. Pigmentation (Figures 158, 159)

An unusual lesion after endotracheal anesthesia is pigmentation of the vocal cords. It is obviously due to the fact that dirt on the surface of the tube has been rubbed into the mucosa (Figures 158, 159).

Fig. 156.

Fibrinous ulcerative laryngitis after intubation. The vocal cords are covered by a thick fibrin membrane and are adherent.

Fig. 157.

Fibrinous ulcerative laryngotracheitis after intubation showing an extensive fibrinous membrane extending from the glottis into the subglottic region. The vocal cords are immobile on both sides due to inflammation.

Fig. 158.

Extensive submucosal pigmentation after endotracheal anesthesia. Particles of dirt were histologically recognizable in the submucosa.

Fig. 159.

Bilateral dark disseminated pigmentation after endotracheal intubation anesthesia.

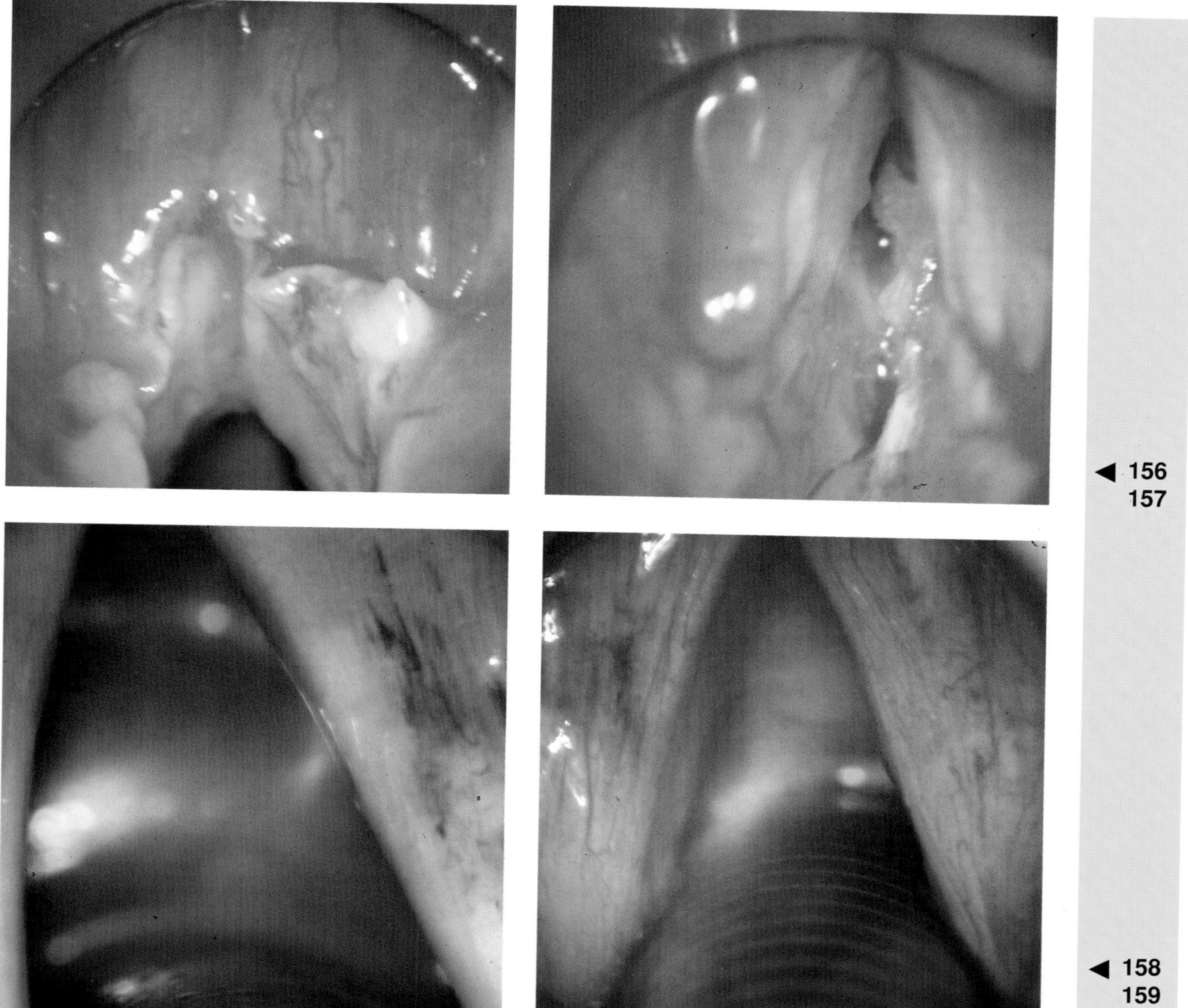

◀ 156
157

◀ 158
159

3. Intubation Granuloma (Figures 160–164)

This lesion can follow endotracheal anesthesia and, rarely, bronchoscopy, but it is usually due to long-term intubation and mechanical respiration. Eighty percent of the patients are women; 75% of the cases are unilateral and 25% bilateral.

Intubation granulomas always arise over the medial surface of the vocal process of the arytenoid cartilage. Unlike contact granuloma, which demonstrates two lips, these lesions are always mushroom-shaped and have a pedicle. The surface is greyish-white or dark red and covered with fibrin and not by epithelium. Most granulomas are detected 2 to 4 weeks after intubation. Granulomas of longer standing can heal spontaneously because the pedicle becomes thinner and the granuloma is finally coughed out. It is probable that many intubation granulomas are coughed out before laryngoscopy is carried out and are therefore not diagnosed.

Treatment is relatively simple and consists of division of the pedicle with scissors. Any remnants of the granuloma are picked off with cupped forceps and the base is carefully coagulated. Recurrence is very unusual. Postoperative speech therapy is not necessary.

4. Traumatic Cysts are described on page 52 (Figure 95)

Fig. 160.

Large intubation granuloma at the typical site over the vocal process of the left vocal cord.

Fig. 161.

Characteristic mushroom-shaped intubation granuloma over the right vocal process.

Fig. 162.

Unusually large mushroom-shaped, fibrin-covered intubation granuloma on the left vocal process.

Fig. 163.

Bilateral intubation granuloma following long-term intubation for drug overdose.

Fig. 164.

Typical mushroom-shaped bilateral intubation granulomas after short-term endotracheal anesthesia.

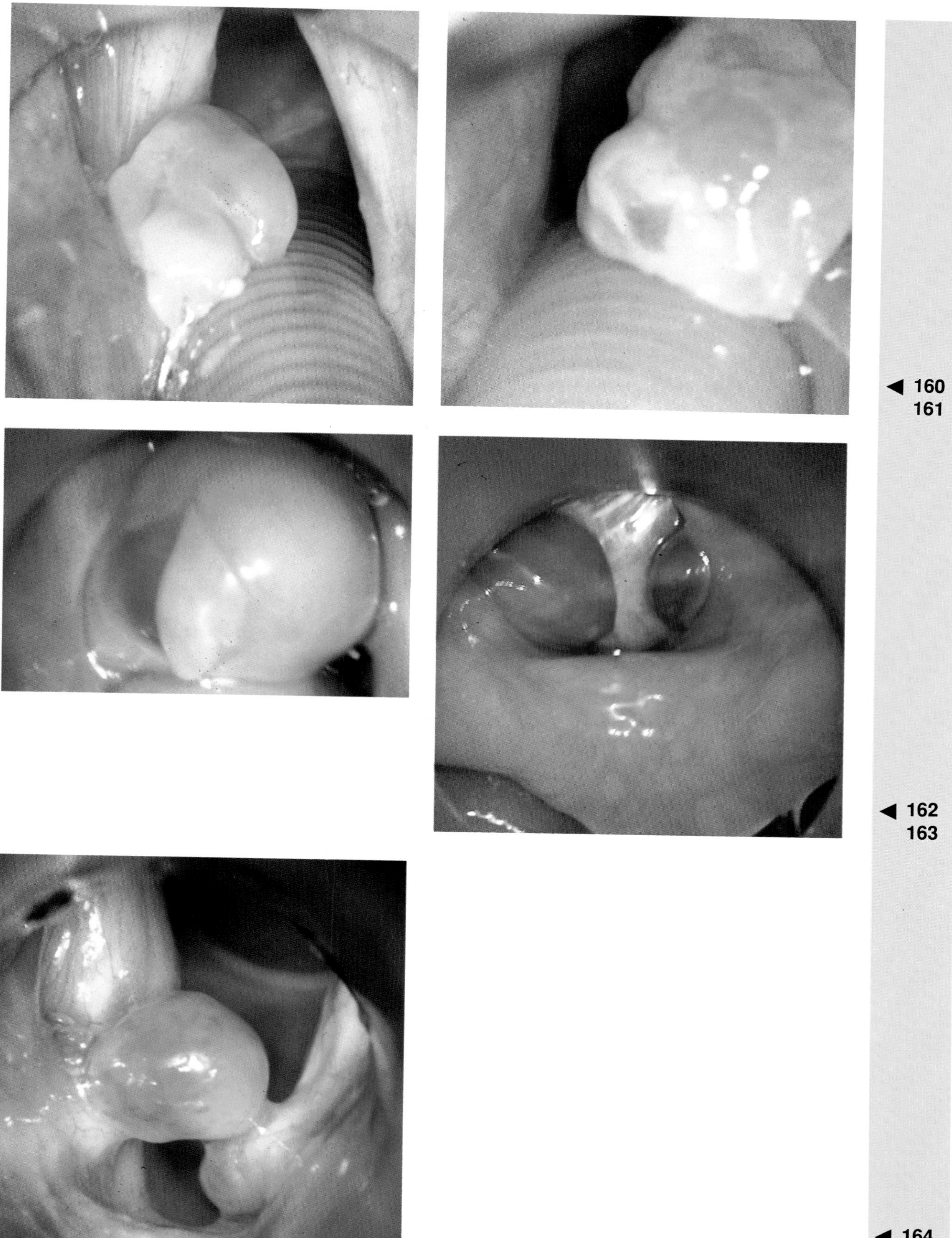

◀ 160
161

◀ 162
163

◀ 164

5. Vocal Cord Synechiae (Figures 165–167)

Intubation may be followed by adhesions affecting the middle and posterior parts of the vocal cords, occasionally the vestibular folds, and very rarely the anterior commissure. Bridge-like bands can be seen uniting the center of the vocal cords or the vestibular folds (Figure 165).

Adhesions between the apices of the vocal process of the two arytenoid cartilages can cause apposition of the entire length of the vocal cords, but sometimes an opening remains anteriorly in the membranous part and posteriorly in the intercartilaginous segment (Figure 166).

This type of adhesion can usually be dealt with by division with scissors. Complete adhesion of the vocal cords along their entire length is very unusual after prolonged intubation (Figure 167).

Fig. 165.

Bridge-like adhesion between the vocal cords after endotracheal anesthesia.

Fig. 166.

Adhesions between the apices of the vocal processes after intubation anesthesia with a narrow glottic chink in front and behind.

Fig. 167.

Complete adhesion of the entire length of both vocal cords after intubation anesthesia.

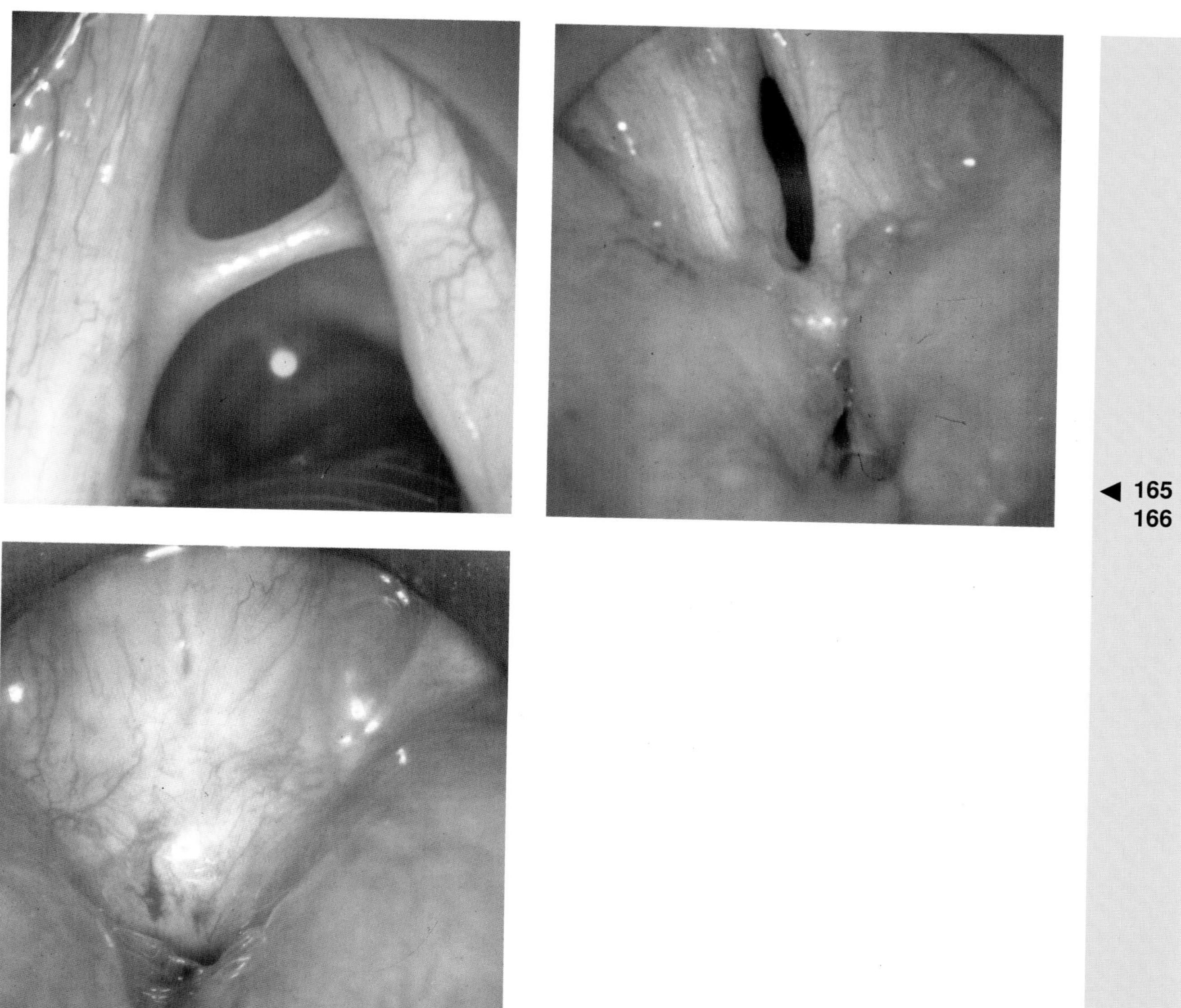

◀ 165
166

◀ 167

6. Subglottic Stenosis (Figures 168–172)

Sadly, subglottic stenosis is still a fairly common complication of endotracheal anesthesia and prolonged intubation, especially in children. This stenosis is particularly likely to follow preexisting mucosal injury, e.g. that due to croup. Two different types can be distinguished, with an intermediate type between them. Diaphragmatic stenoses consist of a membranous ring of scar tissue in the subglottic space (Figures 168, 169, 170). If this ring of scar tissue is not too thick, it can usually be removed completely by endoscopy. The preferred technique for these cases is to puncture the periphery of the stenotic ring at several points with the needle electrode and then to cut out the ring. Sometimes this procedure needs to be repeated. A dilator such as a T-tube should **not** be left in after the operation because this abrades the fresh wound and leads to further scar tissue. Simple dilatation of the annular stenosis, as previously carried out, is unsuccessful.

It is important not to perform surgery until the scar tissue is mature. A lesion that is highly inflamed and consists of granulation tissue has a very high risk of recurrence, and premature, overactive treatment may make matters even worse.

A granuloma noticed immediately after extubation should be removed to avoid a tracheotomy and to prevent the appearance of scar tissue stenosis.

If the subglottic injury extends more deeply and affects the cartilage, chondritis of the cricoid cartilage develops, leading to a rigid circular laryngotracheal stenosis causing partial or complete obstruction. An endoscopic procedure in these cases is nearly always futile (Figures 171, 172).

Fig. 168.

Thin membranous subglottic diaphragmatic stenosis in a child after respiratory treatment.

Fig. 169.

Fresh diaphragmatic stenosis after respiratory therapy. Granulation tissue can still be seen on the posterior edge of the stenosis.

Fig. 170.

Characteristic diaphragmatic stenosis with slightly thickened edges.

Fig. 171.

Funnel-shaped subglottic stenosis at the junction of the larynx and trachea after respiratory therapy.

Fig. 172.

Complete obliteration of the laryngotracheal junction after respiratory therapy.

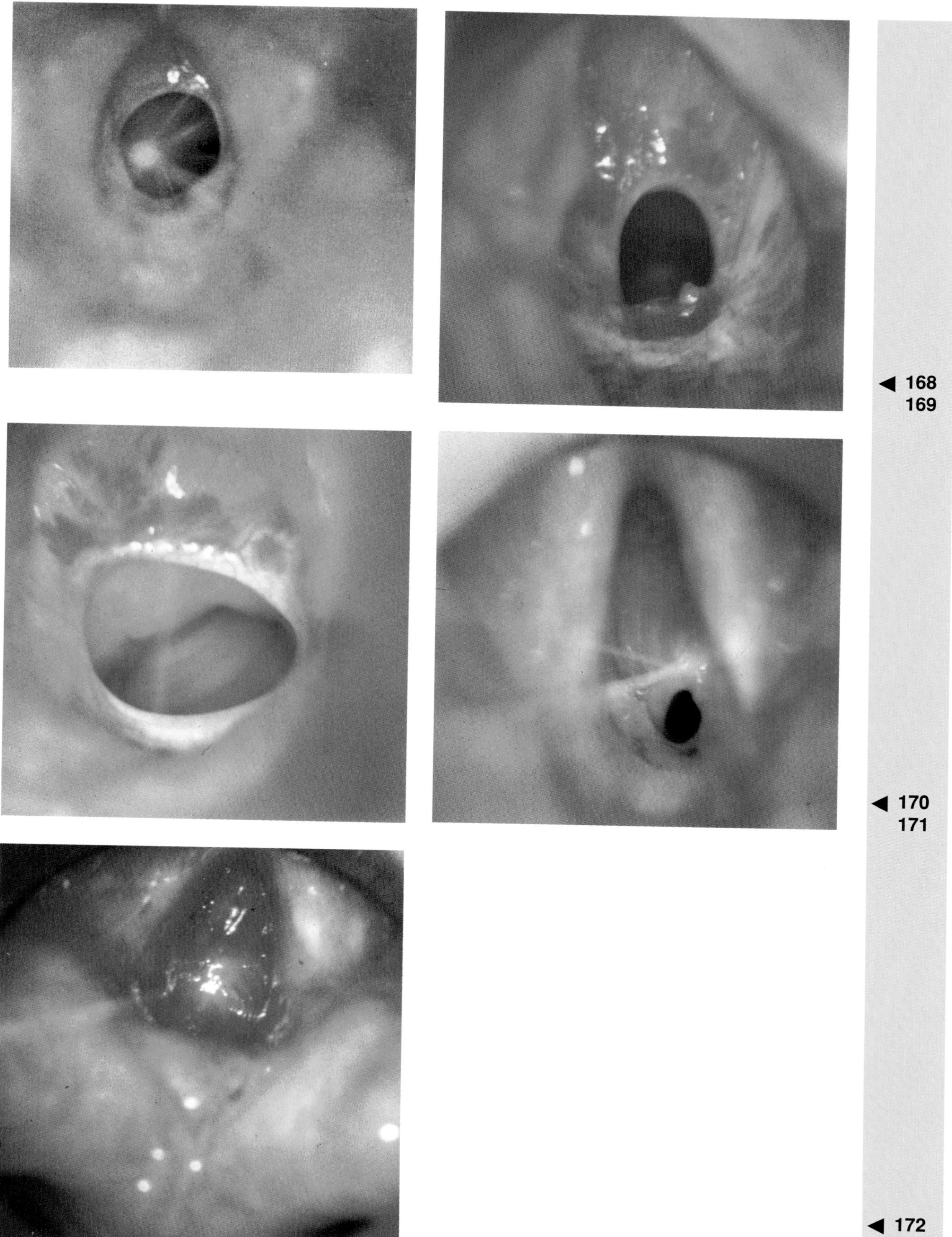

◀ 168
169

◀ 170
171

◀ 172

7. Posterior Scars and Ankylosis of the Cricoarytenoid Joint (Figures 173, 174)

Thick plates of scar tissue often develop on the posterior wall of the larynx from ulcers and granulations that result from abrasion of the plate of the cricoid cartilage by the cuff of an endotracheal tube (Figures 173, 174). Also, the arytenoid cartilages are often found to be ankylosed in the midline, a condition often incorrectly diagnosed as traumatic bilateral recurrent nerve paralysis.

Endoscopic attempts to remove this plate of scar tissue or endoscopic arytenoidectomy to widen the glottis have always been unsuccessful in such cases. Even if arytenoidectomy achieves some widening of the airway, this is usually not enough to allow the patient to be decannulated. A better procedure in these cases is cricoid laminotomy with the interposition of rib cartilage through an external incision.

8. Subluxation of the Arytenoid Cartilage

Subluxation of the arytenoid cartilage after intubation, particularly after crush intubation, is probably overdiagnosed. In all cases that I have seen the arytenoid cartilage was tilted forward and medially and was fixed in this position. Obviously, intubation leads to bleeding into the cricoarytenoid joint and secondary fixation or ankylosis. It is usually futile to attempt to remobilize and reposition the cartilage. If the prolapsed arytenoid cartilage narrows the larynx, the simplest remedy is to resect the apex of the cartilage.

b. Postoperative Granuloma (Figures 175, 176)

Granulomas can follow endoscopic or external laryngeal operations. Some heal or are coughed out, but others persist and grow, leading to dysphonia, and are finally converted into irregular scar tissue (Figures 175, 176). The granulomas arise between 2 and 4 weeks after surgery and are often thought to indicate recurrence of a tumor. It is advisable to remove these granulomas and carefully coagulate their base endoscopically.

Fig. 173.

Plate of scar tissue on the posterior wall of the larynx extending far inferiorly and causing both arytenoid cartilages to adhere.

Fig. 174.

Asymmetrical plate of scar tissue on the posterior wall of the larynx extending from left to right and fixing the arytenoid cartilage.

Fig. 175.

Postoperative granuloma after endoscopic operation for carcinoma-in-situ.

Fig. 176.

Postoperative subglottic granuloma after partial laryngectomy for carcinoma.

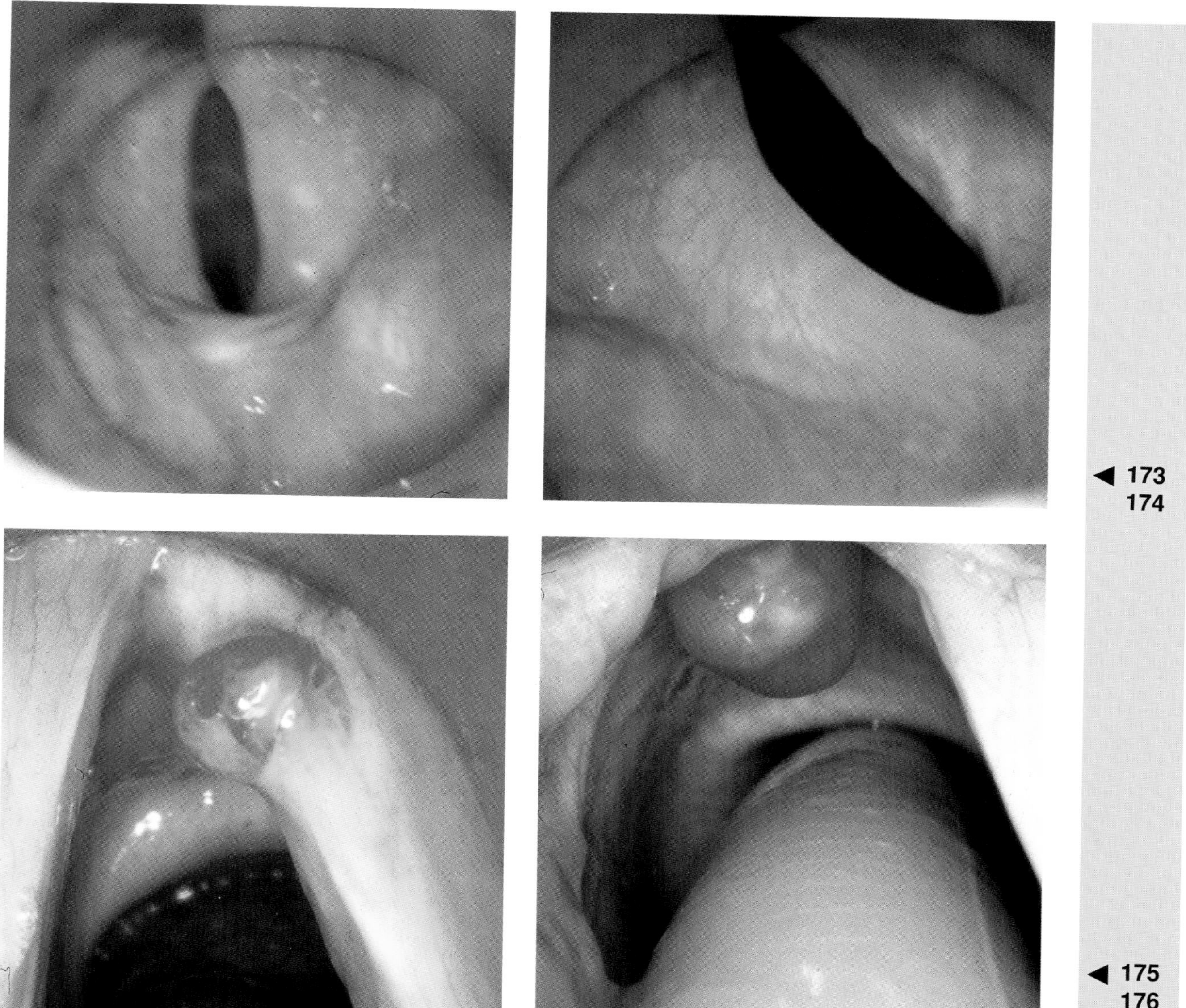

◀ 173
174

◀ 175
176

c. Anterior Synechiae (Figures 177–179)

Anterior synechiae may arise after endolaryngeal surgery, after laryngeal fractures or fissures, and especially after thyrotomy or cordectomy (Figures 177–179).

The preferred treatment is to divide the synechiae, if necesary at several sittings, to restore the acute angle of the anterior commissure. The mucosal defects must be as small as possible. A notch on the vocal cord due to the traction of the scar tissue can often be seen. Sadly, endoscopic division of synechiae is often followed by recurrence. Sometimes it is only possible to remove the synechiae partially or to narrow them, because their anterior segment is relatively thick and extends inferiorly. In such cases, treatment may be attempted by the technique described by Haslinger in 1923, according to which a separator (keel) is fixed with a translaryngeal suture. But this method may also be followed by recurrences. Mucosal grafts fixed with tissue glue are usually rejected.

d. Mucoceles After Partial Laryngectomy (Figures 180, 181)

A mucocele of the saccule may sometimes follow cordectomy or hemilaryngectomy, particularly if the saccular mucosa is not completely removed or everted. These mucoceles (also termed internal laryngoceles) present as a swelling of the affected area. A part of the vestibular fold is resected, both as treatment for the lesion and to exclude a concealed recurrence of tumor.

Fig. 177.

Adhesions between the vocal cords after removal of papillomas.

Fig. 178.

Extensive plate of scar tissue after operation for bilateral vocal cord nodules.

Fig. 179.

Adhesions of the vocal cords are particularly common after repeated removal of juvenile laryngeal papillomas.

Fig. 180.

Mucocele or cyst in the left vestibular fold after hemilaryngectomy.

Fig. 181.

Large mucocele after hemilaryngectomy almost completely obstructing the glottis.

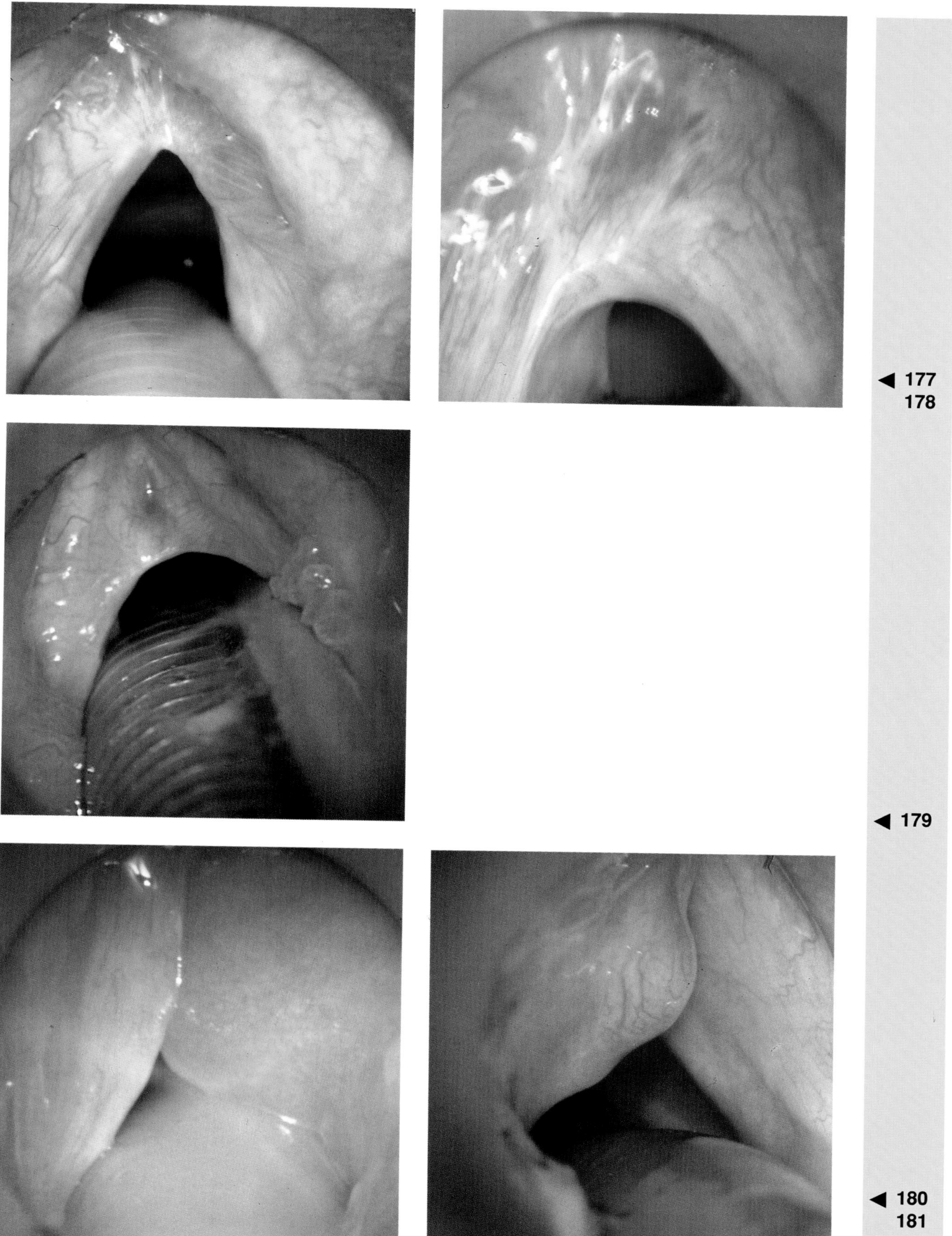

◀ 177
178

◀ 179

◀ 180
181

4. Congenital Anomalies

a. Congenital Web (Figures 182, 183)

This very unusual lesion is extremely difficult to deal with by endoscopy because as a rule only the posterior edge of the web is thin and transparent, whereas in front it consists of a wide plate of connective tissue extending downward to the cricoid cartilage, often in association with an anomaly of the cartilage (Figures 182, 183).

Division of the thin part of the web during endoscopy is usually enough to improve the airway. Complete removal of a congenital web would require thyrotomy and mucosal repair, but this operation has not been tried extensively and its results are difficult to predict.

b. Cleft Larynx (Figures 184, 185)

This extremely rare disease is characterized by a cleft in the plate of the cricoid cartilage through which a mucosal fold prolapses and narrows the glottis (Figures 184, 185). Palpation of this mucosal fold reveals the underlying defect in the cartilage. Endoscopic resection of this anomaly is not possible. I have only seen two adult patients, both of whom were treated by lateral pharyngotomy, careful separation of the wall of the esophagus from the overlying intralaryngeal mucosa, and resection of the superfluous mucosa. These patients often suffer aspiration, although of usually minor degree.

c. Intralaryngeal Ectopic Thyroid Tissue

This unusual lesion presents as a greyish-red, smooth swelling posterolaterally at the junction of the larynx and the trachea. Biopsy can lead to brisk bleeding. Treatment consists of thyroidectomy and resection of the intraluminal tumor via an external approach, as used for thyroid carcinoma invading the larynx.[47, 54]

d. Glottic Sulcus

These rare furrows of varying depth in the vocal cords I have never treated by surgery. Bouchayer has stated that this lesion is of congenital origin.[3, 4]

Fig. 182.
Congenital laryngeal diaphragm.

Fig. 183.
Extensive congenital laryngeal diaphragm.

Fig. 184.
Posterior cleft larynx showing the mucosa of the inter-arytenoid region bulging forward.

Fig. 185.
Posterior cleft larynx showing the wall of the esophagus and the posterior wall of the larynx prolapsing like a sac into the arytenoid region.

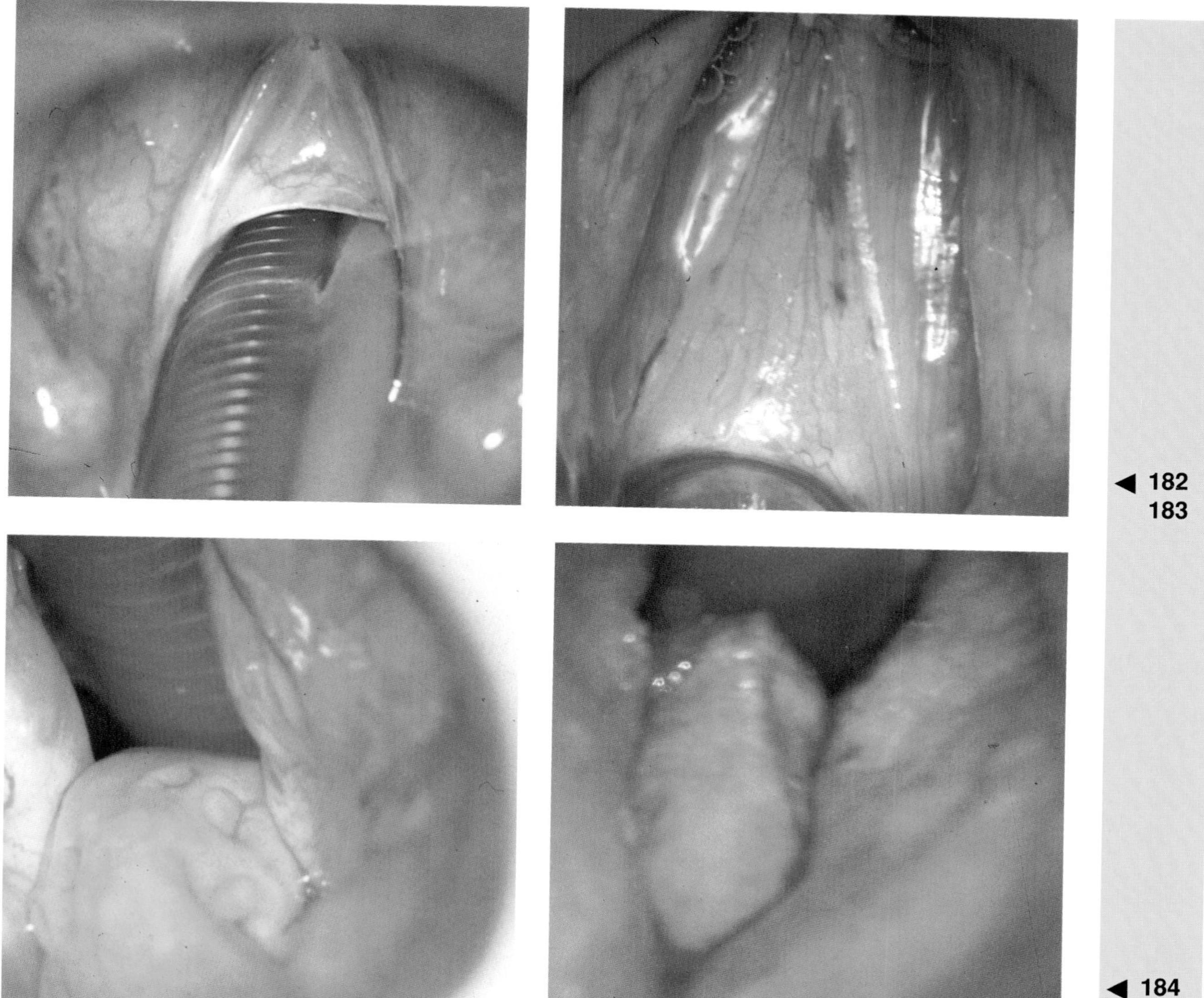

◀ 182
183

◀ 184
185

5. Endoscopic Surgery of Laryngeal Paralysis

For unilateral paralysis in the paramedian positon I prefer medialization of the vocal cord using Peyer's trapdoor thyroplasty or an extraperichondrial implantation of cartilage as described by Meurman.[35] I have no experience with the injection of artificial material such as silicone and so forth for the augmentation of a paralyzed vocal cord and will not discuss these techniques further.

None of the many attempts to restore the function of the recurrent laryngeal nerve by anastomosis has yet given reproducible results in bilateral paralysis of the recurrent laryngeal nerve. Indeed, it is technically impossible to reunite the antagonistic fibers for the abductor and adductor muscles, which are integrated in one nerve. The alternative is performing one of the various external or endoscopic procedures on the laryngeal skeleton or muscles to widen the glottic chink. The disadvantage of all these procedures is that the wider the glottis, the better the breathing, but the worse the voice. Endolaryngeal arytenoidectomy for expansion of the glottic chink was described by Thornell in 1948. Endolaryngeal microsurgery has allowed the development of a technically easier procedure in which the vocal cord is thinned by partial submucosal removal of the muscles and by vertical division of the conus elasticus, a step that produces further widening of the glottic chink.[36] This procedure has been widely adopted and further modified, for example by hitching the posterior end of the vocal cord to the vestibular fold, by closing the surgical defect with tissue glue rather than sutures, and by excision of the arytenoid cartilage using the laser. By 1988 I had done 230 procedures, and almost all (98%) of these patients have been decannulated. This procedure is technically not easy, but its advantage is that widening of the glottis can be tailored to the patient's weight and the size of the larynx by individualized thinning of one vocal cord. In a few cases the glottic chink was too wide and the voice therefore poor, but in general the voice is better than that which can be achieved by external lateral fixation of the cord.

The results of arytenoidectomy are much less satisfactory for bilateral ankylosis of the cricoarytenoid joint resulting from external trauma, prolonged intubation, irradiation of the thyroid gland or larynx, or polyarthritis. In such cases the procedure of choice is a laminotomy of the cricoid plate and interposition of a piece of rib cartilage into the posterior wall of the larynx through an external approach.

The indication for endolaryngeal arytenoidectomy is bilateral paralysis of the recurrent laryngeal nerve after thyroid surgery, usually for a recurrent goiter. About 90% of our cases were women. Surgery should not be undertaken until at least 6 months after the thyroidectomy because many patients achieve spontaneous partial or complete recovery. However, none of a small series of patients with bilateral paralysis of the recurrent laryngeal nerve due to an epidemic of influenza followed up for a year achieved spontaneous recovery. An immediate arytenoidectomy can be carried out if both recurrent laryngeal nerves are divided at an operation for thyroid carcinoma. In a few cases the paralysis is incomplete on one side, and the operation should then be carried out on the completely paralyzed side. Movements in the region of the arytenoid cartilage produced by motor fibers of the superior laryngeal nerve that supply the ventricularis muscle and the small muscle in the aryepiglottic fold can mimic incomplete paralysis. Preoperative investigation should include pulmonary function tests and radiographs of the trachea. A proven tracheal stenosis must be dealt with first and the larynx operated on at a later date; otherwise the end result may be a patient condemned to a permanent tracheostomy with an even worse voice due to his widened glottic chink, if the tracheal stenosis later proves to be beyond correction. Many patients only come in for surgery after bilateral paralysis has been present for many years. Many of these women have become inactive because of the chronic hypoxia and have become obese, so that the larynx is relatively small in comparison with their body weight. These patients should lose weight before an operation to widen the glottis. The age of the patient does not need to be considered before embarking upon arytenoidectomy; decannulation can be achieved in adolescents and in patients over 80 years old. One contraindication to endolaryngeal arytenoidectomy is the tendency to form keloid or hypertrophic scars. These patients are probably better dealt with by an external laterofixation without opening the mucosa of the larynx.

Some patients have already undergone an external laterofixation. An endoscopic procedure usually shows that the suture used for laterofixation has cut out, allowing the glottis to narrow again. Satisfactory widening can be achieved by complete removal of the arytenoid, and especially by vertical division of the conus elasticus. Some patients who had submitted to endolaryngeal surgery elsewhere were found to have granulations and scar tissue due to splinters of the arytenoid cartilage. In all of these cases division of the conus elasticus had been omitted.

I have no personal experience with the endoscopic operation of infants with congenital paralysis of the recurrent laryngeal nerves.

The operation always begins with a tracheotomy if the patient does not already have one. The tracheotomy can be used to resect a recurrent goiter and to correct the scar after thyroidectomy. Arytenoidectomy without tracheotomy is technically possible but places the patient at risk.

A large caliber (size B) laryngoscope is used. Dissection is carried out using small scissors and a knife, and hemostasis is achieved with the microcoagulator. Catgut on a small diameter needle is used for the suture. The needle is usually round, and it is helpful to flatten its body with a diamond burr to facilitate grasping by the needle holder. A powerful forceps is useful for removing the arytenoid cartilage from the joint once it has been mobilized.

Figure 186 shows the steps of the procedure

At the end of the operation a flexible cuffed plastic tracheostomy tube is left in place to prevent aspiration in the event of a secondary hemorrhage. The cuff can usually be released a few hours after the operation. Bleeding is very unusual but can be dangerous if it arises from the superior laryngeal artery. This artery can sometimes be seen in the depth of the wound after removal of the arytenoid cartilage and in such cases should be ligated as a precaution. Later secondary hemorrhage from this artery is dealt with by reintubation, packing of the trachea, and ligation of the artery after external exposure. A few patients suffer persistent edema of the arytenoid region for days or even weeks. Marked edema may follow intensive use of electrocoagulation.

If wound healing proceeds normally, the patient is fitted with a valved tracheostomy tube 6–8 days after the operation. If respiration is then satisfactory, the tracheostomy tube is corked, at first during the day and then at night also. The tracheostomy tube can be removed as soon as the patient is able to climb stairs with the tube occluded. We have usually been able to decannulate most patients between 8 and 14 days after the operation. Daily inhalation therapy is prescribed until the tracheostomy tube is removed. A few patients must be decannulated gradually over a long period because they are anxious and frightened of choking, even though the glottis is of satisfactory width. Some patients can be allowed home with the tracheostomy tube in place and be readmitted several weeks later for decannulation. Large granulomas should be removed, although most of them will be coughed out spontaneously.

Several years later a few patients develop a submucosal edema resembling Reinke's edema of the opposite, non-operated side. These patients can be satisfactorily treated by excising a strip of this tissue to restore a glottis of satisfactory width.

The voice can often be improved by speech therapy begun only after complete healing has been achieved.

186 ▶

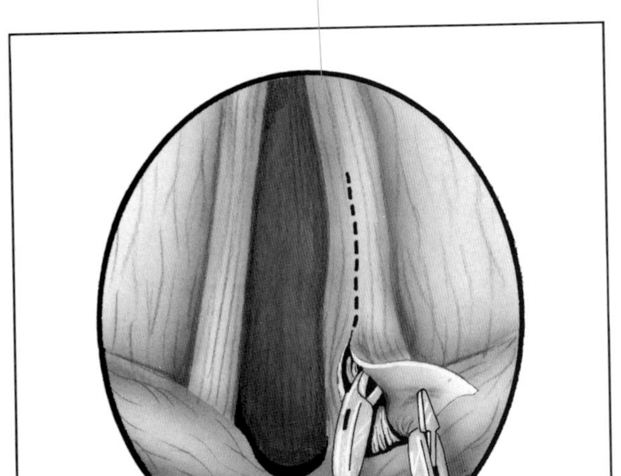

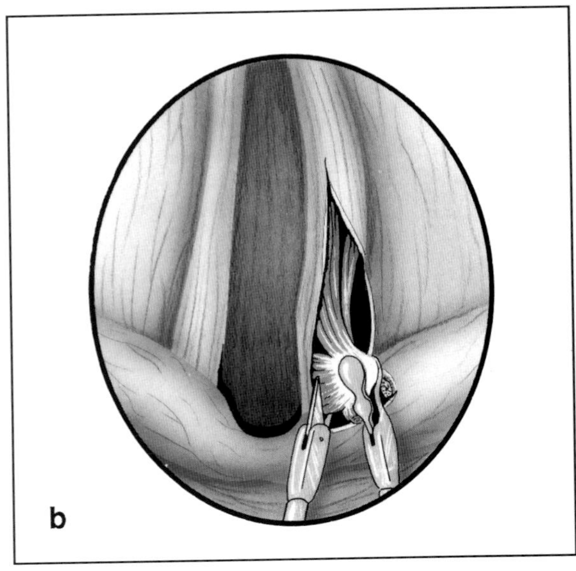

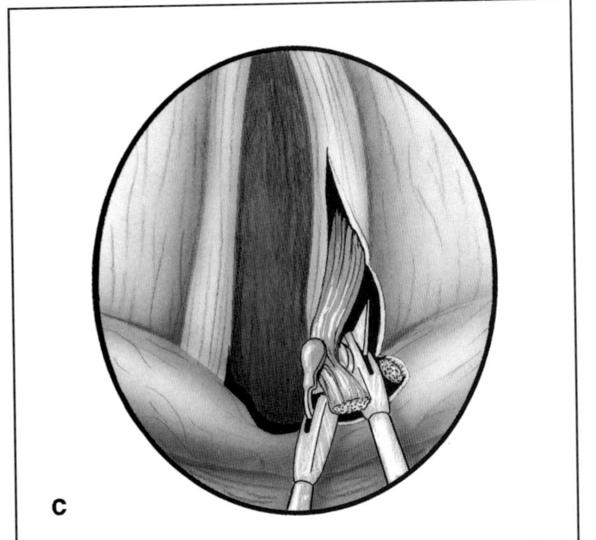

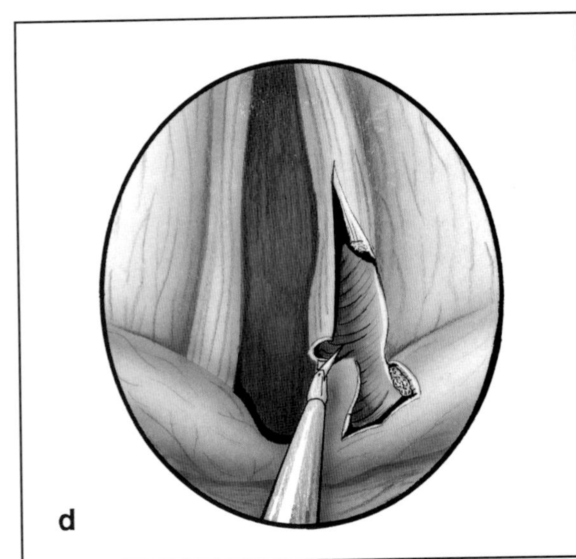

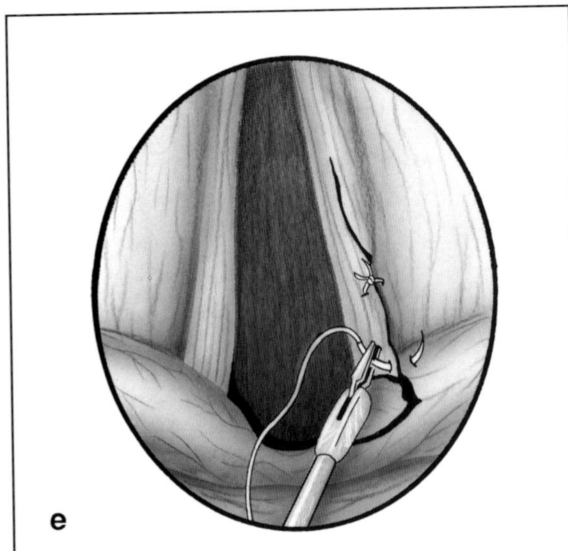

Fig. 186 a.
Excision of a triangular piece of epithelium.

Fig. 186 b.
Dissection of the arytenoid cartilage.

Fig. 186 c.
Partial excision of the vocalis muscle.

Fig. 186 d.
Vertical incision into the conus elasticus.

Fig. 186 e.
Wound closure by sutures.

6. Laryngeal Tumors

a. Squamous Cell Carcinoma and Premalignant Lesions

The development of microlaryngoscopy was stimulated by the wish to inspect the larynx under magnification, with special emphasis on the early recognition of premalignant states and carcinomas. Of all vocal cord carcinomas detected in the Marburg Clinic over the past 15 years 63% were in the stages of carcinoma-in-situ or microinvasive carcinoma (T_1), thanks to the improved health education of the general population and the increasing awareness of general practitioners, but undoubtedly also to the fact that microlaryngoscopy was performed on all patients with even the slightest suspicion of a tumor.[12] In addition there were numerous cases of benign keratoma, a tumor that is, however, a facultative premalignant lesion. Supraglottic and hypopharyngeal carcinomas do not produce the significant symptom of hoarseness, and most still present in an advanced stage with regional lymph node metastases.

Routine use of microlaryngoscopy over the past 30 years has taught us the great variability in the microlaryngoscopic appearances of squamous cell carcinoma and its precursors. A further important field for the use of microlaryngoscopy is its value in monitoring after partial laryngectomy or irradiation of laryngeal carcinoma.

Even if the microlaryngoscopic appearances are highly characteristic, histologic analysis is always required to distinguish between simple keratosis, carcinoma in situ, and microinvasive and macroinvasive carcinoma. The histologic subclassification of epithelial hyperplasias and premalignant lesions of the larynx was elaborated in the first years of microlaryngoscopy. With the passage of time therapy became more and more important in addition to diagnosis. Endolaryngeal microsurgery developed in parallel with microlaryngoscopy and made it possible to take a biopsy accurately from specific parts of the lesion. The next step was functional conservative microsurgical endoscopic resection of benign keratomas and senile papillomas. Finally came systematic endoscopic resection of premalignant lesions and squamous cell carcinomas, which has been used often and successfully over the last decade in selected cases.

Definitions and Terminology of Epithelial Lesions.[26, 42] Unfortunately no uniform terminology for epithelial lesions of the larynx has yet become generally accepted, so that a multitude of terms is applied to lesions that are sometimes the same and sometimes different. Many names are based solely on external appearances, such as leukoplakia, erythroplakia, hyperkeratosis, pachydermia, verruca, and papilloma. These macroscopic descriptions convey nothing of the degree of differentiation of a tumor or its prognosis and should therefore be replaced by terms based on the microscopic structure, as follows:

Grade I (Figure 187). The squamous epithelium is usually hyperplastic, acanthotic, and covered by a keratinous layer of varying thickness. The increased growth rate of the thickened epithelium manifests itself by verrucae, papillae, and villi. However histologic examination shows regular stratification and differentiation of cells in all layers, and absence of nuclear atypia and usually of mitoses. (Synonymous terms are simple atypia and simple dysplasia.)

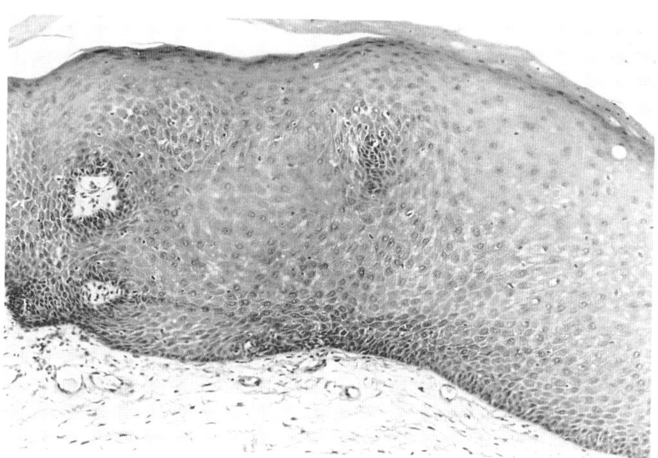

Fig. 187.

Grade I squamous cell hyperplasia (so-called keratosis). The squamous epithelium shows acanthosis and wart-like proliferations which are covered by horny layers. Internally, however, the epithelium shows regular differentiation without stratification disorders or nuclear atypia.

Grade I epithelial hyperplasia is usually an expression of inflammation due to chronic hyperplastic laryngitis or contact granuloma. A further form is that arising within an otherwise healthy thin epithelium, characterized by a slightly projecting, papilliferous or villous surface and termed benign keratoma, or senile papilloma if appropriate. These are true benign tumors. A keratoma of histologic Grade I is usually benign and remains so. Since these cases cannot be classified without a biopsy, and since excisional biopsy alters the natural history of the disease, it is impossible to assess the frequency of progression to carcinoma. However, it may be assumed that in the course of time a few cases will develop into carcinoma, as has been shown by a study of senile papillomas. Therefore these lesions should be regarded as facultative premalignant disorders.

Grade II (Figure 188). Grades I, II, and III can be distinguished solely by microscopy. Grade II lesions show occasional nuclear atypia and locally circumscribed abnormalities of differentiation within the epithelium. However, these lesions are not pronounced enough to be classified as premalignant (Grade III), nor are they still entirely benign (Grade I). Therefore these cases fall into the "wait and see" group, or Grade II. The experienced pathologist repeatedly sees cases that he is unable to classify with certainty as either entirely benign or already premalignant, and that are therefore better classified in an intermediate group. For the clinician the diagnosis of a Grade II lesion demands a particularly careful follow-up.

Grade III (Figure 189). I prefer the term carcinoma in situ for these cases, even if the abnormal maturation of the epithelium and the nuclear dysplasia do not extend to all the epithelial layers. Carcinoma-in-situ shows the same variations of differentiation as a full-blown carcinoma, that is, well-differentiated squamous cell and undifferentiated basal cell forms in addition to moderately matured transitional forms. Grade III is a collective term for lesions that other authors have called increased atypical epithelium, severe dysplasia, carcinoma-in-situ, carcinoma stage 0, intraepithelial carcinoma, etc. It is not justifiable to distinguish between carcinoma-in-situ that is characterized by cellular atypia in all the epithelial layers, and high grade atypia or dysplasia with differentiation in the upper epithelial layers only. The difference between these lesions is only a matter of degree, and their prognosis is similar. All Grade III lesions are likely to progress to an infiltrating carcinoma. Since it is impossible to know whether the lesion will progress rapidly to infiltration or whether this event will be delayed for years, all these lesions should be treated immediately as an early carcinoma.

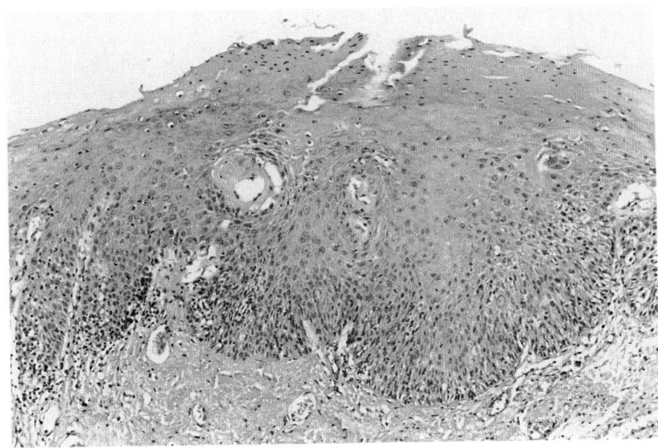

Fig. 188.

Grade II squamous cell hyperplasia showing thickened squamous epithelium with slightly abnormal stratification and a few scattered atypical nuclei.

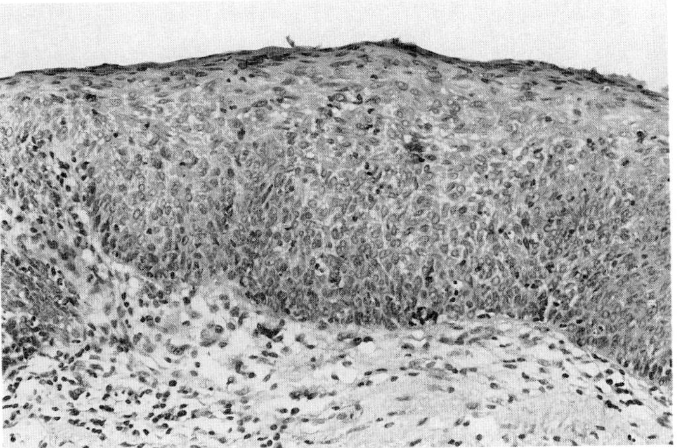

Fig. 189.

Grade III squamous cell hyperplasia or carcinoma-in-situ, showing coarse abnormalities of differentiation and stratification and nuclear atypia in almost all layers of the epithelium.

Microcarcinoma and Microinvasive Carcinoma. The vocal cord is one of the few parts of the body where very small carcinomas develop relatively often. Microcarcinoma describes a superficial carcinoma with a maximum size of 10 x 10 x 3 mm, and microinvasive carcinoma a tumor that has not yet infiltrated the muscle of the vocal cord. These terms have been borrowed from gynecological pathology.[31] These small tumors are of course relatively easy to treat, and there is a high probability of cure. However, this favorable state of affairs is due to their minimal extent and the absence of metastases, and not to a lesser degree of malignancy compared with macroinvasive cancers.

The previously popular concept that every squamous cell carcinoma arises from a premalignant lesion is erroneous. I have seen several carcinomas, particularly those arising from chronic laryngitis, that arose directly from the basal epithelial layers and infiltrated deeply, whereas the overlying epithelium showed normal maturation and stratification and concealed the menacing lesion lying more deeply. It is impossible to say how many carcinomas arise directly from the basal epithelial layers and are thus not accessible to early diagnosis with currently available methods, and how many arise from a preexisting carcinoma-in-situ that has been present for a varying period of time

Microlaryngoscopic Aspects of Premalignant Lesions and Carcinoma (Figures 190–242).

Grade I keratoma and also Grade II lesions arise almost exclusively from the membranous segment of the vocal cords (Figures 190–200). Their surface is uneven, sometimes quite markedly papilliferous, and always covered with a keratin layer of varying thickness. Tumors with a pronounced villous surface and very marked keratinization are termed senile or adult papillomas. The surrounding epithelium is thin and transluscent and the underlying capillaries can be clearly seen. The size of the keratoma varies from 2 to 3 mm to large tumors occupying the entire vocal cord. The size of the tumor does not necessarily correlate with its differentiation. Palpation of a keratoma always clearly shows that it is freely movable along with the surrounding epithelium over the underlying muscle of the vocal cord, so that it can be freed easily from the vocal ligament by dissection in Reinke's space.

Fig. 190.

Benign keratoma in the center of the left vocal cord, appearing as a small papillary and keratinized tumor. Histologic grade I.

Fig. 191.

Benign keratoma of the left vocal cord with a contact reaction on the right side. Small keratinized papillary tumor. Histologic grade I.

Fig. 192.

Benign keratoma, histologic grade I, lying close to the anterior commissure on the right side.

Fig. 193.

Benign keratoma extending on the subglottic surface of half the right vocal cord. Histologic grade II.

Fig. 194.

Benign keratoma of the left vocal cord. The epithelium is opaque, but the thickened area is relatively sharply demarcated with papillae at the center. Histologic, grade I.

Fig. 195.

Benign keratoma grade I with a small tumor in the center and a sharply demarcated thickening of the surrounding epithelium. Contact reaction on the right vocal cord.

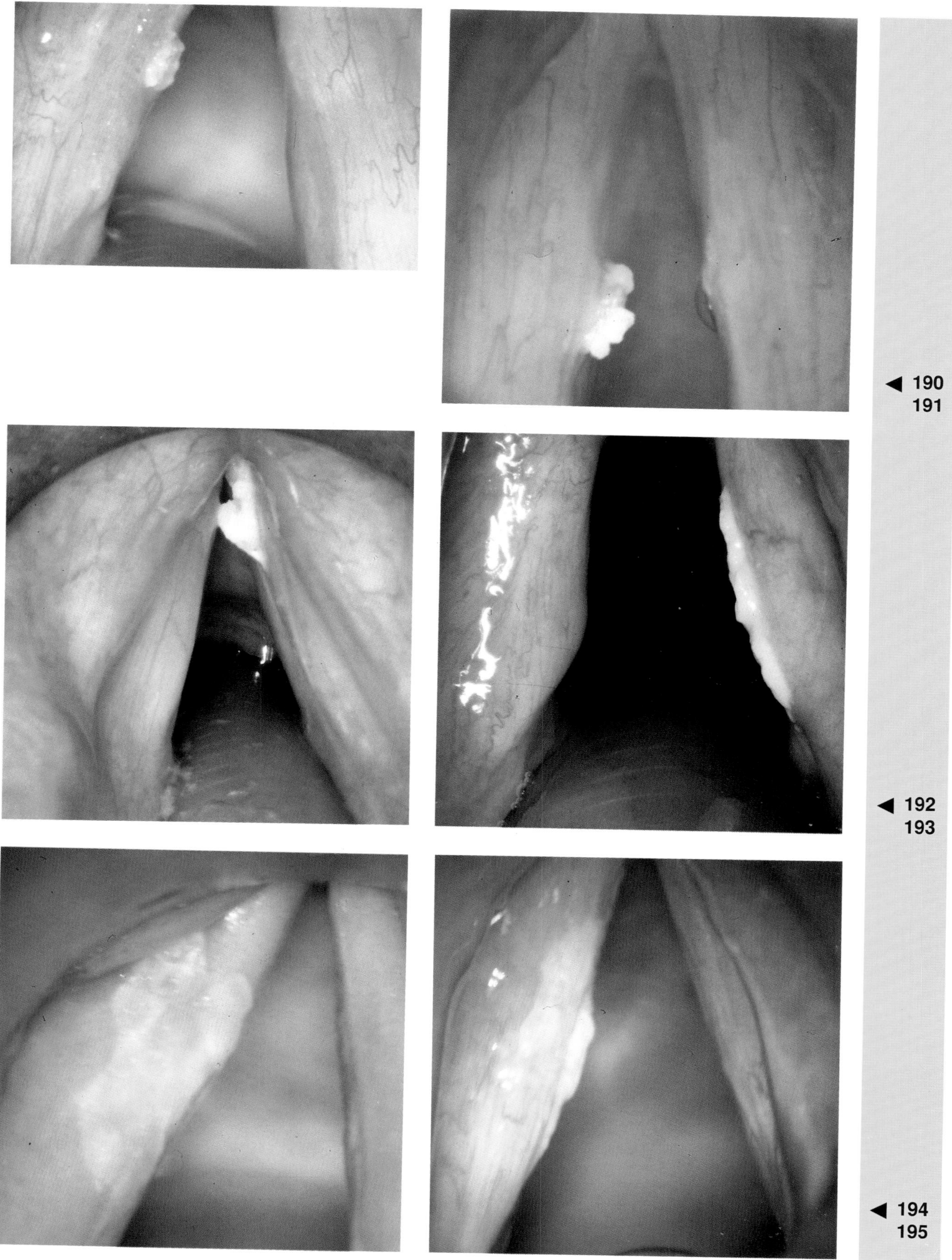

◀ 190
191

◀ 192
193

◀ 194
195

Extensive villous keratoses are often difficult to distinguish from verrucous acanthosis.

About two-thirds of cases of carcinoma-in-situ demonstrate keratinization of widely varying extent of the surface (Figures 201–206); sometimes the reddish granular epithelial surface is covered with scattered individual flakes of keratin, and at other times entirely by a thick keratinous layer. About one-third of cases are not keratinized, and their surface is finely granular or papilliferous (Figures 207–210). It should be noted that erythroplakias of this type are not found in Grade I lesions. An important indication of premalignancy or malignancy is the presence of atypical U-shaped, corkscrew-shaped, or hook-shaped capillaries of varying caliber that can be recognized on the nonkeratinized surface of the tumor (Figures 207–213).

Fig. 196.

Papillary keratoma (senile papilloma) of the left vocal cord, histologic grade II.

Fig. 197.

Senile papilloma of the left vocal cord showing sharply demarcated, papillary, keratinizing surface (histologic grade I).

Fig. 198.

Large senile papilloma of the right vocal cord, histologic grade I.

Fig. 199.

Senile papilloma of the left vocal cord with keratinized surface. This tumor can only be distinguished from carcinoma by histologic study.

Fig. 200.

A large senile papilloma of the right vocal cord, histologic grade I.

Fig. 201.

Small warty carcinoma-in-situ of the right vocal cord.

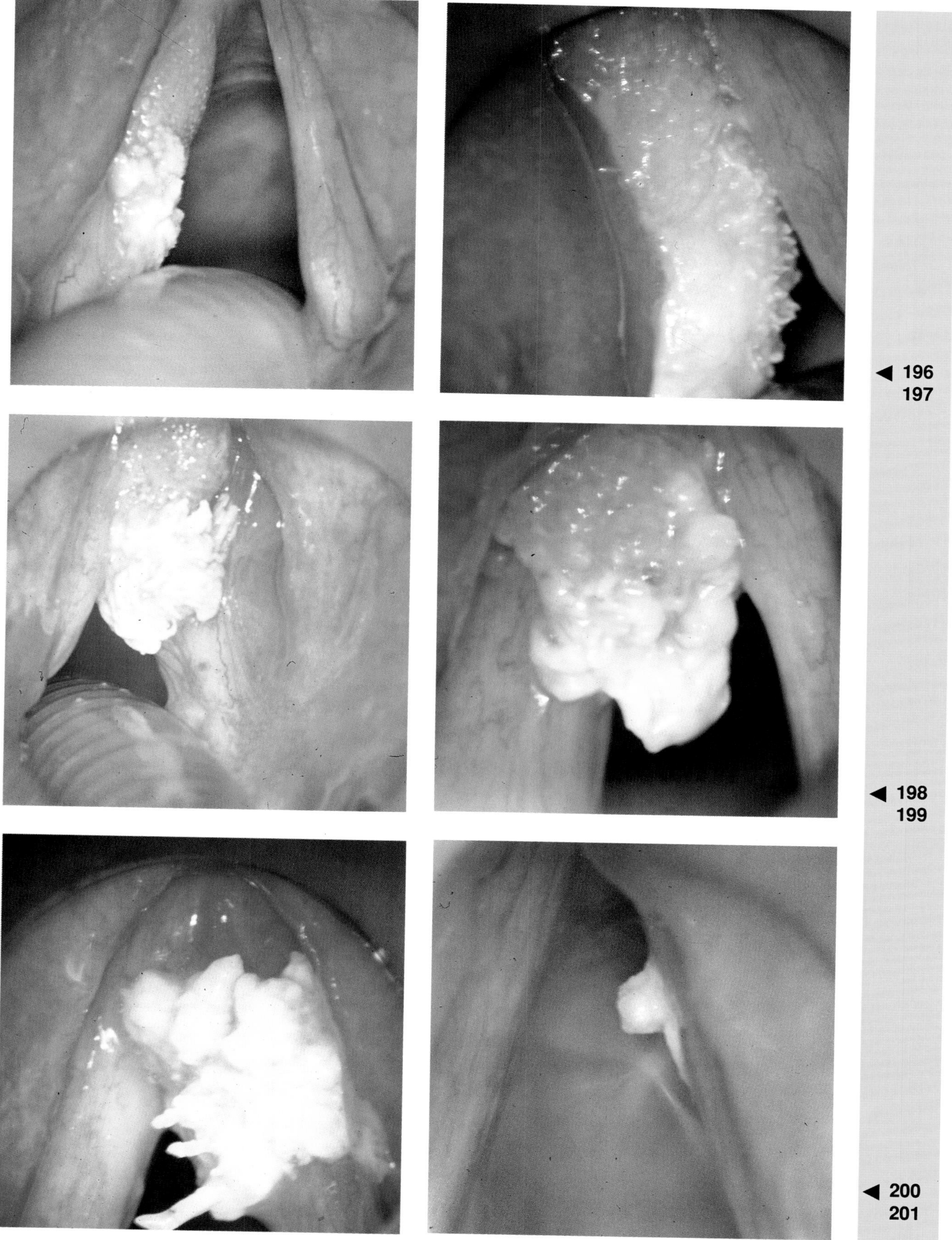

◀ 196
197

◀ 198
199

◀ 200
201

Fig. 202.

Carcinoma-in-situ of the left vocal cord with a small satellite focus.

Fig. 203.

Carcinoma-in-situ of the left vocal cord in an exophytic but not yet infiltrating form.

Fig. 204.

This carcinoma-in-situ mainly arose on the subglottic surface of the vocal cord but has extended over almost all the entire membranous part of the vocal cord.

Fig. 205.

Same case as in Figure 204. Rotation of the vocal cord shows the warty keratinized carcinoma-in-situ.

Fig. 206.

Very extensive carcinoma-in-situ of the left vocal cord. Despite the extent of the tumor serial sections do not yet show infiltration.

Fig. 207.

Carcinoma-in-situ of the left vocal cord with pronounced polypoid appearance. A few atypical capillaries can be seen on the surface.

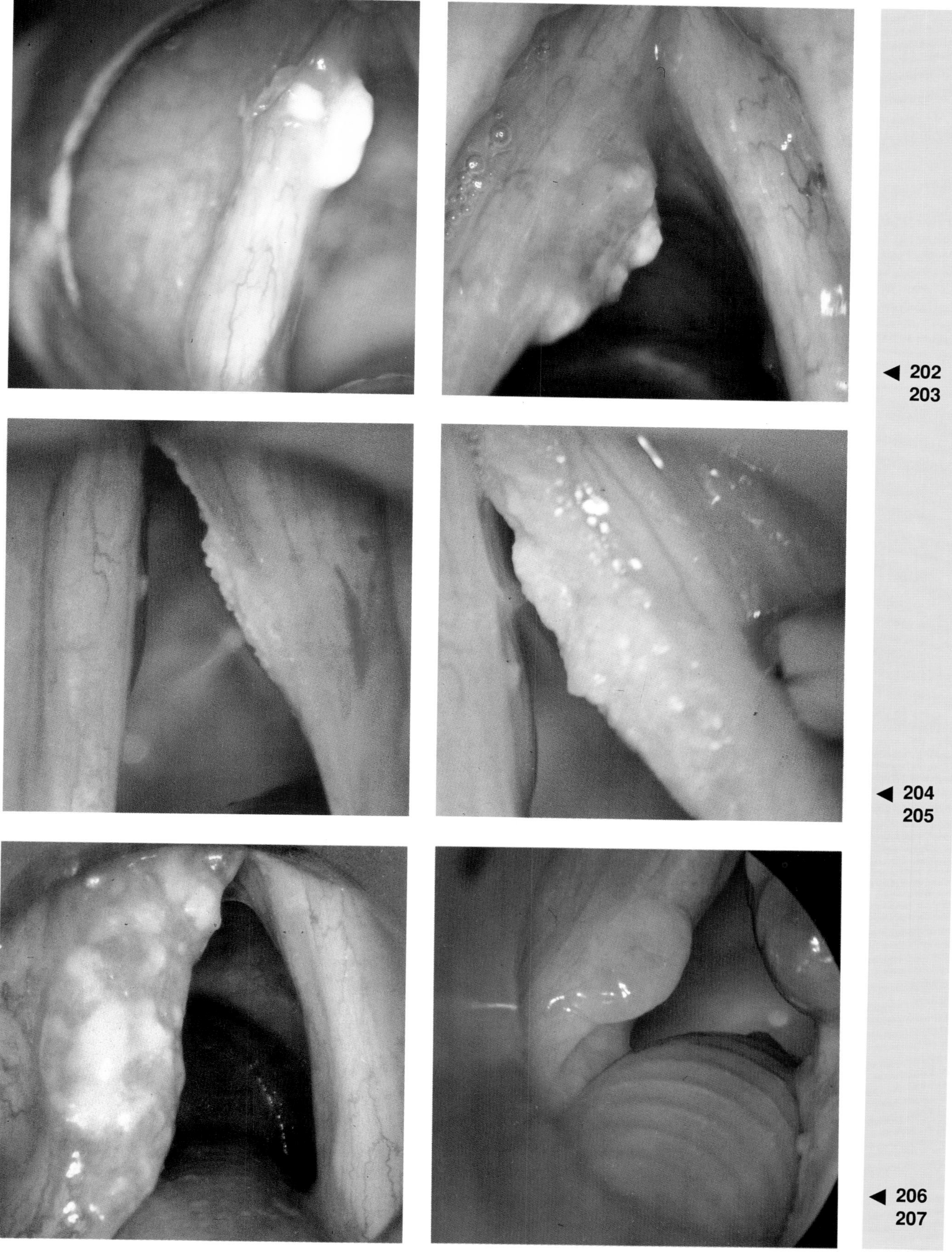

◀ 202
203

◀ 204
205

◀ 206
207

Fig. 208.

Carcinoma-in-situ of the right vocal cord at an unusual site at the junction of the squamous and respiratory epithelium in the floor of the ventricle. The surface of the tumor is covered by numerous atypical capillaries.

Fig. 209.

Carcinoma-in-situ of the anterior third of the left vocal cord showing an occasional slight thickening of the epithelium and fine granularity, but no evidence whatever of keratinization.

Fig. 210.

Small carcinoma-in-situ of the left vocal cord without keratinization. The right vocal cord shows reactive edema.

Fig. 211.

Carcinoma-in-situ of the left vocal cord showing a small circumscribed lesion resembling a polyp.

Fig. 212.

Small carcinoma-in-situ lying close to the anterior commissure on the left side. Only slight redness and thickening of the epithelium can be seen.

Fig. 213.

Carcinoma-in-situ of the entire right vocal cord. The surface of the epithelium is relatively smooth; the epithelium is occasionally thickened and reddened due to increased capillarity.

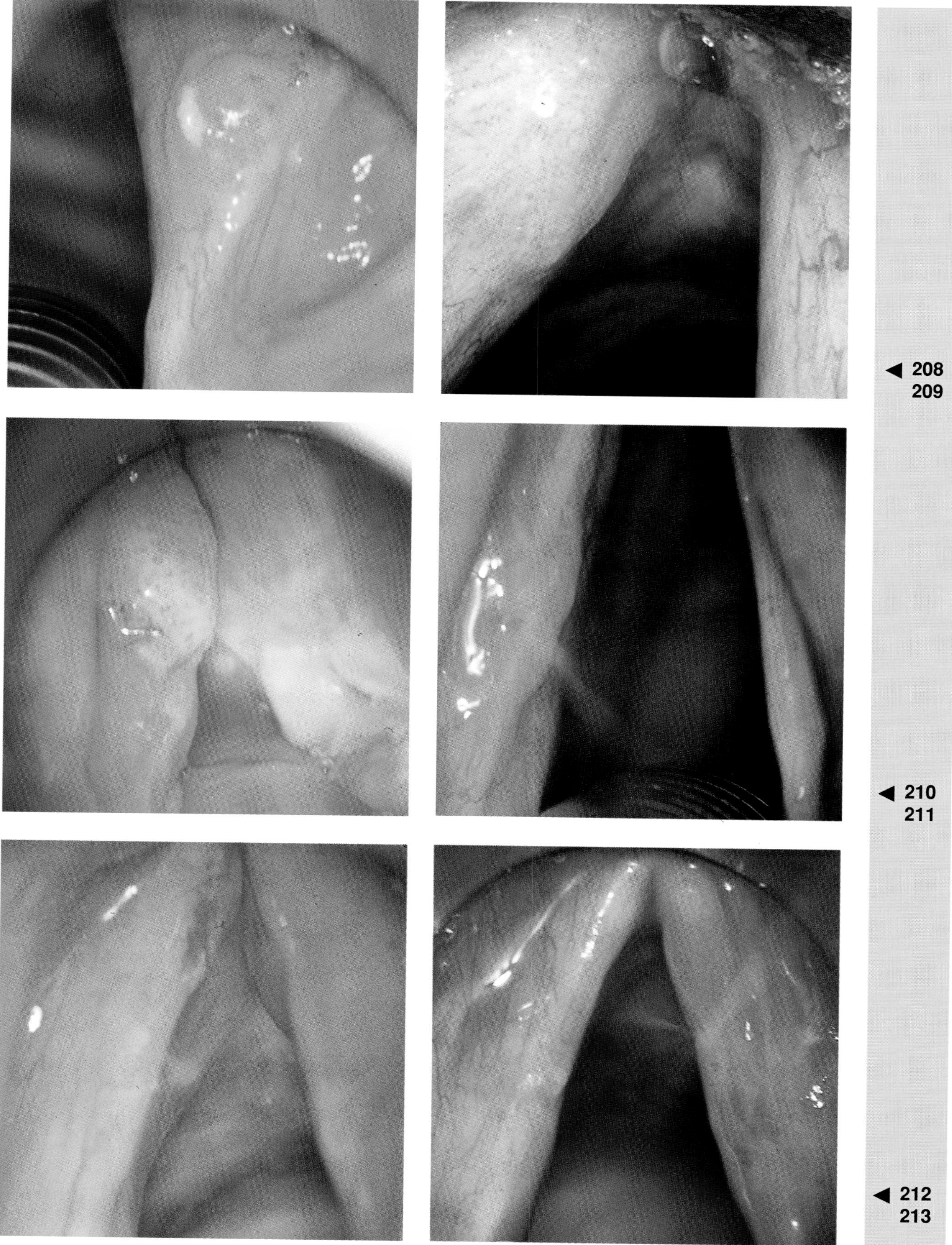

◀ 208
209

◀ 210
211

◀ 212
213

Like carcinoma of the vocal cord, carcinoma-in-situ is often bilateral (Figures 214, 215) and arises from an extensive field of cancerization extending over both vocal cords (Figures 216, 217). In addition to this superficially spreading carcinoma, multiple separate foci that merge later in the disease are also quite common (Figures 218, 219).

Fig. 214.

Primary bilateral carcinoma-in-situ. The tumor occupies the entire vocal cord and the anterior third of the right cord. On the left side a large flat ulcer is seen on the surface of the tumor.

Fig. 215.

Extensive carcinoma-in-situ of the left vocal cord. A grade II epithelial lesion on the right vocal cord.

Fig. 216.

Superficially spreading carcinoma (carpet carcinoma) on both vocal cords. The tumor was still at the in-situ stage at all points.

Fig. 217.

Bilateral malignant change (cancerization) of both vocal cords. Microinvasive carcinoma was already present at a few sites, but the remainder of the tumor was at the in-situ stage.

Fig. 218.

Multicentric carcinoma-in-situ. The tumor on the left vocal cord is of the nonkeratinized type. On the right vocal cord there is a second carcinoma-in-situ separated by a strip of as yet unthickened epithelium.

Fig. 219.

Multicentric carcinoma-in-situ. On the left side there is a small carcinoma-in-situ and a further isolated focus of carcinoma-in-situ is seen in the center of the right vocal cord.

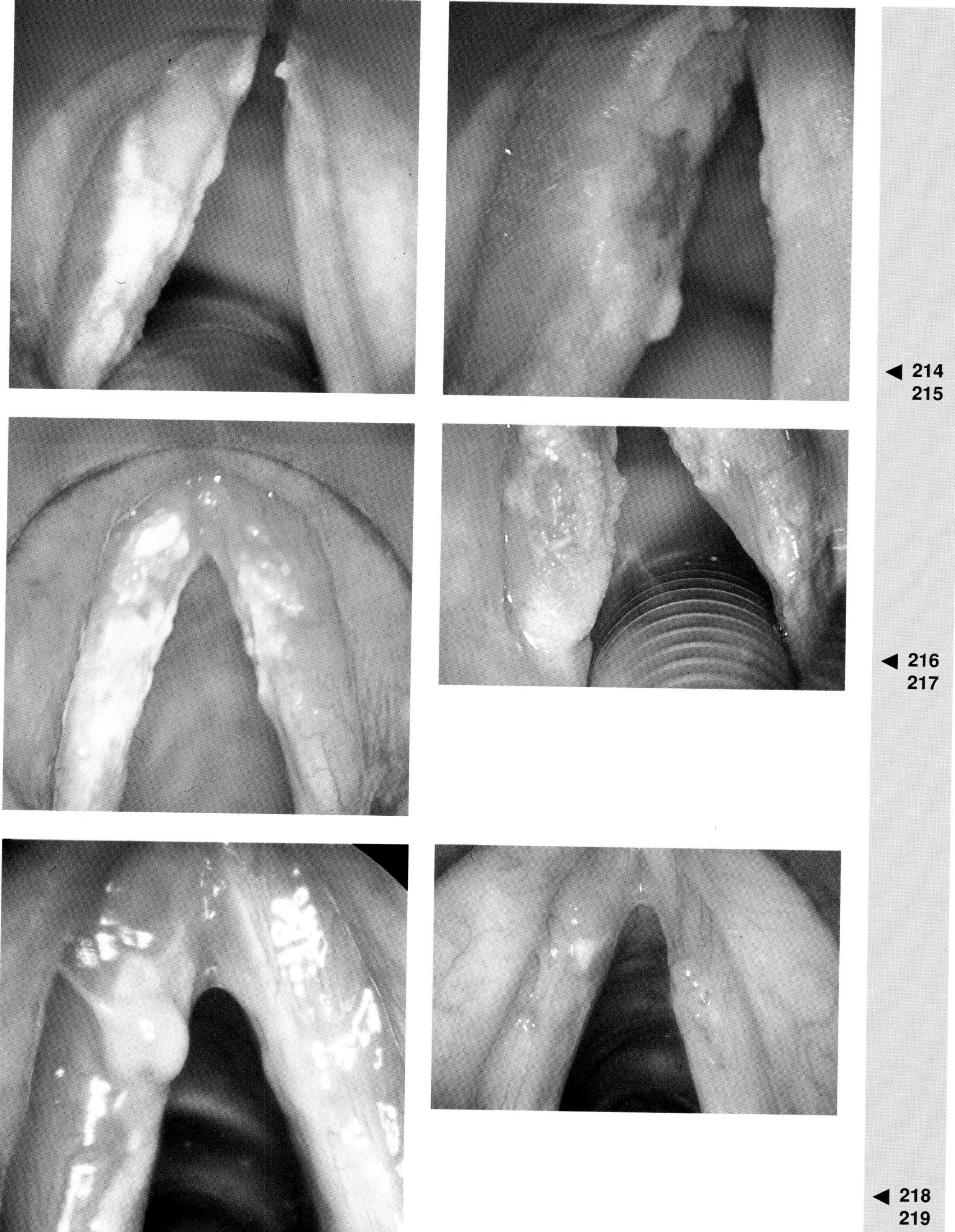

◀ 214
215

◀ 216
217

◀ 218
219

Carcinoma-in-situ and microinvasive carcinomas are readily movable over the soft muscular body of the vocal cord. Important indications of deeper invasion include immobile areas of the tumors, hard areas in the vocal cord, or nodular swellings; superficial ulceration of a small tumor also indicates infiltration. The superficial blood supply becomes insufficient at the point where the tumor infiltrates, causing necrosis (Figures 220, 223).

In the case of carcinoma it is particularly important to assess the superficial extent of the tumor as accurately as possible so that the question of partial resection of the larynx can be decided. The infraglottic segment of the larynx, the entrance to the ventricle, and the vestibular folds must be examined with a 30° or 70° telescope (page 9).

Fig. 220.

Microcarcinoma of the left vocal cord with central retraction as a sign of infiltration.

Fig. 221.

Microcarcinoma of the right vocal cord. The vocal cord is reddened so that the warty, sharply circumscribed tumor on the subglottic surface is more clearly seen.

Fig. 222.

Microcarcinoma of the left vocal cord showing superficial capillary atypia.

Fig. 223.

Polypoid microcarcinoma of the right vocal cord with a small central ulcer.

Fig. 224.

A pT1 vocal cord carcinoma with superficial infiltration arising from the anterior half of the right vocal cord.

Fig. 225.

Histologic category pT2 vocal cord carcinoma infiltrating into muscle.

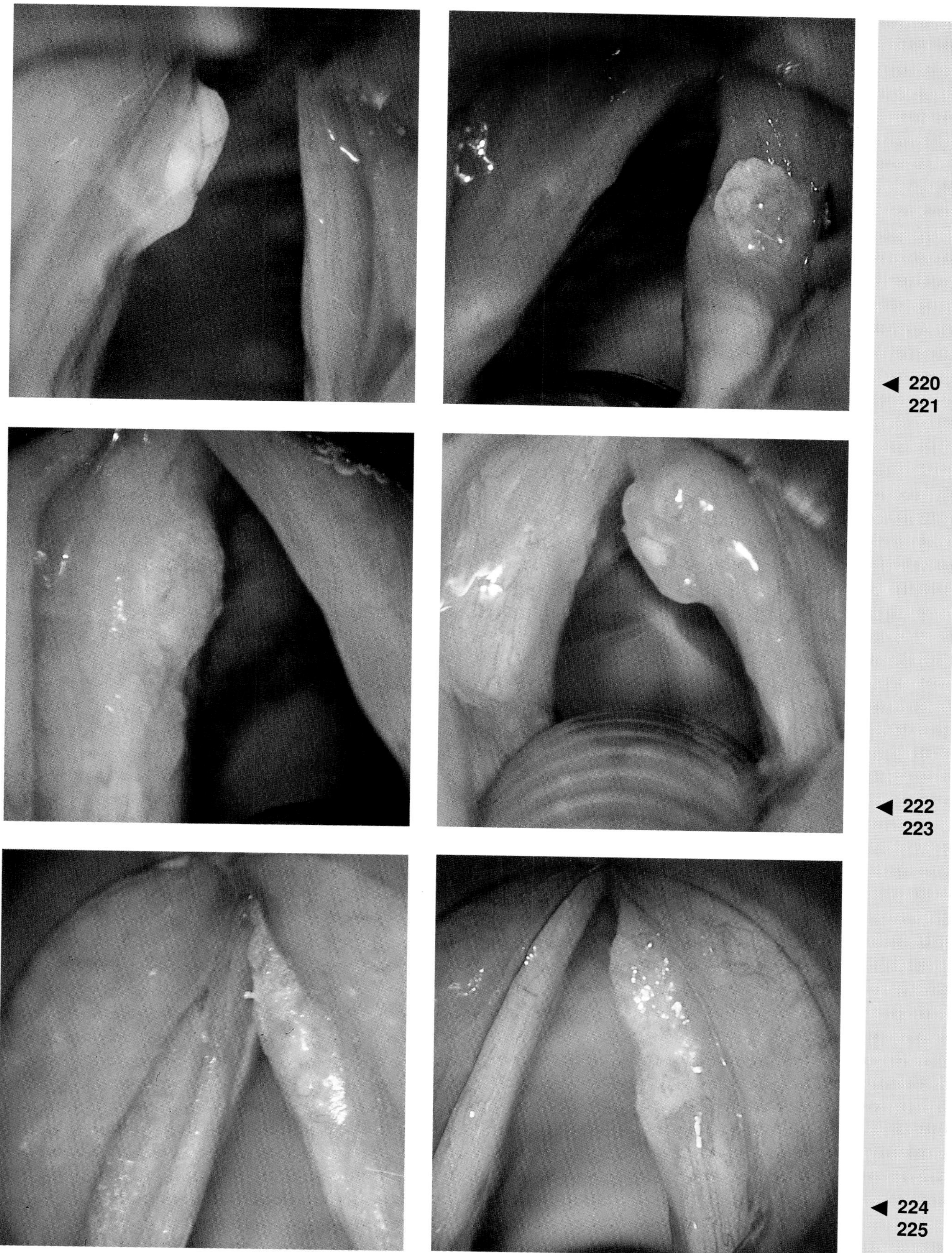

◀ 220
221

◀ 222
223

◀ 224
225

The appearance of a large carcinoma is usually so typical that the diagnosis can be made with great certainty even before histologic examination of a biopsy (Figures 224–233). However, it must not be forgotten that tuberculosis can occasionally mimic a laryngeal carcinoma. Furthermore, there are some large carcinomas that have already deeply infiltrated, although the changes on the surface of the vocal cord are difficult to recognize. These unusual cases are characterized by red or yellowish discoloration of the vocal cord epithelium and a few atypical capillaries, so that these tumors can be very easily overlooked (Figure 234). Well-developed polypoid exophytic tumors with the laryngoscopic appearance of a polyp or granuloma are also relatively unusual (Figures 235, 236), and histologic studies show many of these cases to be pseudosarcomas or carcinosarcomas.[29]

Fig. 226.

Category pT2 vocal cord carcinoma extending over the entire length of the left vocal cord to the vocal process.

Fig. 227.

Subglottic vocal cord carcinoma at the anterior commissure. The tumor can only be seen by parting the two vocal cords. Histologic examination showed a pT2 tumor.

Fig. 228.

Primary bilateral vocal cord carcinoma at the anterior commissure.

Fig. 229.

Carcinoma of the anterior commissure spreading upward between the vestibular folds to the petiole.

Fig. 230.

Bilateral keratinizing vocal cord carcinoma with a deep ulcer anteriorly on the right side. Histologic examination showed a pT3 tumor.

Fig. 231.

Extensive endolaryngeal, so-called transglottic carcinoma involving the vestibular folds and vocal cords.

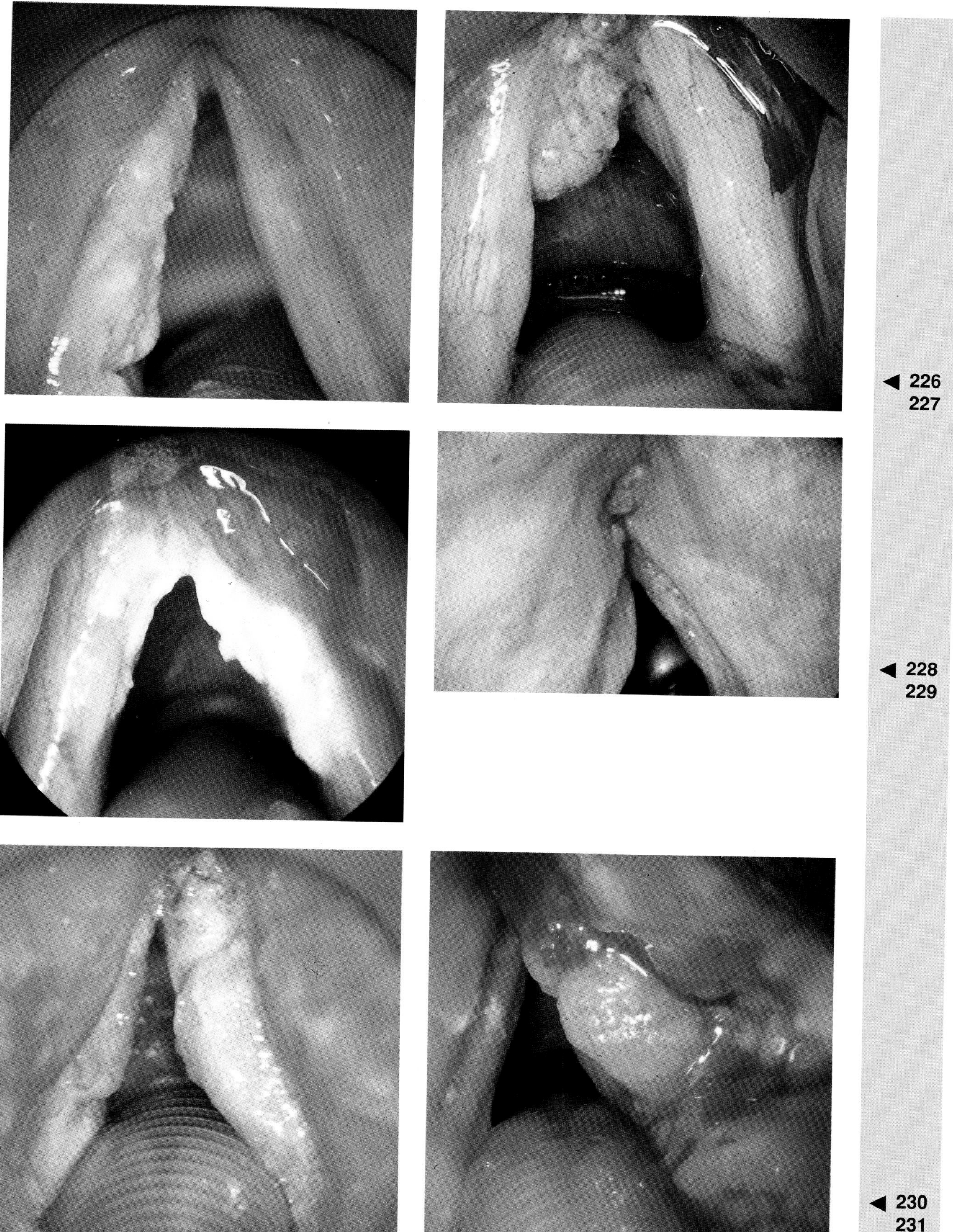

◀ 226
227

◀ 228
229

◀ 230
231

Supraglottic carcinomas are viewed tangentially at microlaryngoscopy, and it is much more difficult to assess their superficial extent accurately (Figures 237–239). Tumors lying on the laryngeal surface of the epiglottis, in particular, can be concealed by the laryngoscope. Supraglottic carcinomas are best demonstrated by withdrawing the laryngoscope slowly – possibly placing it in the vallecula – and then pushing the epiglottis posteriorly by external pressure so that the tumor is pressed into the laryngoscope and may be more clearly seen; its extent can then be measured using a small mirror, or, if preferred, a 70° endoscope.

Hypopharyngeal carcinomas, on the other hand, are usually readily seen with the laryngoscope (Figures 240, 241). A large laryngoscope must be used and, on occasion, a long scope to expose the inferior extension of a carcinoma of the piriform sinus or postcricoid space into the cervical esophagus (Figure 242).

Fig. 232.

A pT3 vocal cord carcinoma invading the ventricle.

Fig. 233.

Large vocal cord carcinoma mainly lying beneath the glottis. The lesion was a nonkeratinizing papillary tumor.

Fig. 234.

A tumor infiltrating deeply into the vocal cord musculature but with a mainly smooth surface of thickened epithelium with increased capillary atypia.

Fig. 235.

Polypoid carcinoma arising from the left ventricle on the left vestibular fold. Histologic examination showed a carcinosarcoma (pseudosarcoma).

Fig. 236.

Pronounced polypoid nonkeratinizing tumor of the right vocal cord and vestibular fold. Histologic examination showed a carcinosarcoma.

Fig. 237.

Carcinoma of the angle of the epiglottis and the vestibular fold on the left side with marked keratinization.

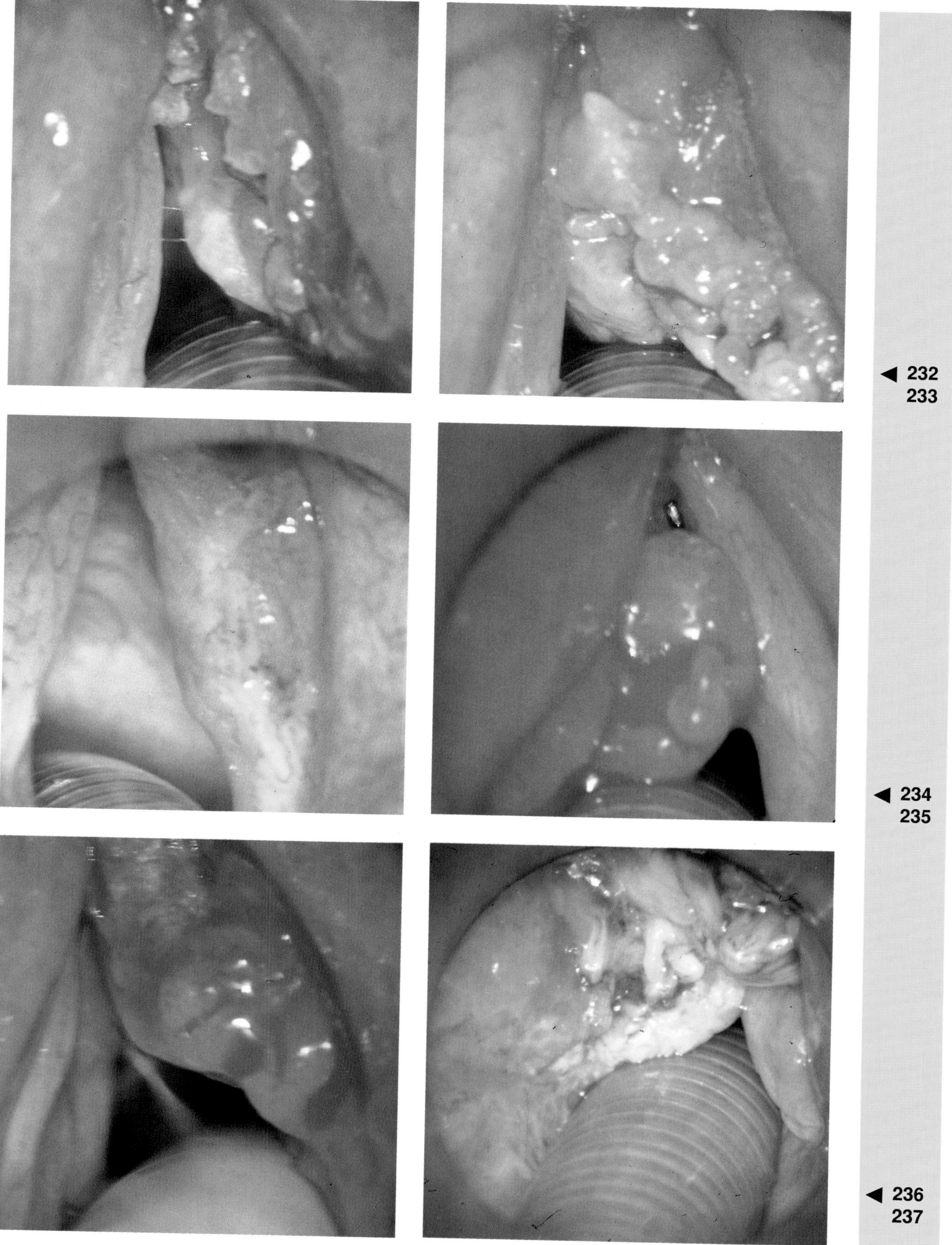

◀ 232
233

◀ 234
235

◀ 236
237

b. Endoscopic Surgery for Premalignant Lesions and Laryngeal Carcinoma

The great advantage of endolaryngeal microsurgery is that it allows a biopsy to be taken from a selected site and a piece of tissue to be removed without crushing it. Thus, tissue may be removed from the center of the tumor or from suspect areas at the edge of the tumor. It is also important to ensure that pieces of the vocal cord muscles or the vocal ligaments are not removed unnecessarily. In a few cases it may be difficult to find tumor tissue, for example, after irradiation therapy complicated by persistent edema and inflammation. In such cases islets of carcinoma sometimes lie more deeply and can only be exposed by a mucosal incision. A wide-bore needle may be useful for finding tumor in the vallecula, the base of the tongue, or the depth of the vestibular fold. Although positive findings with a wide-bore needle do indeed indicate the presence of tumor, negative findings cannot be assumed to exclude the presence of tumor.

It may be necessary to debulk a laryngeal carcinoma to provide a satisfactory airway, either for palliative reasons or to pre-empt the need for a tracheotomy. The high-frequency electrosurgical unit is very useful, allowing large parts of the tumor to be pared off without causing brisk bleeding.

I try to resect small tumors of the vocal cord (and the rare small tumors of the supraglottic region) immediately and in one piece, if this is technically possible. The tumor is circumscribed and freed from the underlying layers, taking great care not to damage the vocal ligament or the laryngeal musculature. If histologic examination shows that the lesion is a Grade I or II keratoma or senile papilloma, excisional biopsy is the definitive treatment. Even if examination shows a carcinoma-in-situ or a small carcinoma, this procedure is also the definitive treatment, provided that histologic study shows that the tumor has been completely removed.

The earlier controversy about the safety of endoscopic resection of vocal cord carcinoma has currently been resumed, because microlaryngoscopy has made it technically possible to remove a tumor accurately in one piece from the vocal cord.[33] Since the introduction of the laser into endoscopic surgery, several laryngologists have now started to carry out endolaryngeal resection of even extensive tumors.

The most important prerequisite for the success of endoscopic resection of a vocal cord carcinoma is careful and conservative assessment. This operation puts both the patient's life and his voice at stake and should therefore only be carried out by a laryngologist experienced in both diagnostic and therapeutic microlaryngoscopy.

Fig. 238.

Extensive nonkeratinizing epiglottic carcinoma.

Fig. 239.

Warty, nonkeratinizing carcinoma of the epiglottis. The epiglottis has been elevated with the tip of the laryngoscope to provide a better view of the tumor.

Fig. 240.

Small carcinoma of the pirifom sinus with numerous atypical capillaries.

Fig. 241.

Extensive hypopharyngeal carcinoma extending from the piriform fossa to invade the posterior wall of the pharynx.

Fig. 242.

Postcricoid carcinoma. View into the esophageal inlet.

Fig. 243.

Erythema and edema of the vocal cords after radiotherapy. The swollen vestibular folds are blanched by the pressure of the laryngoscope.

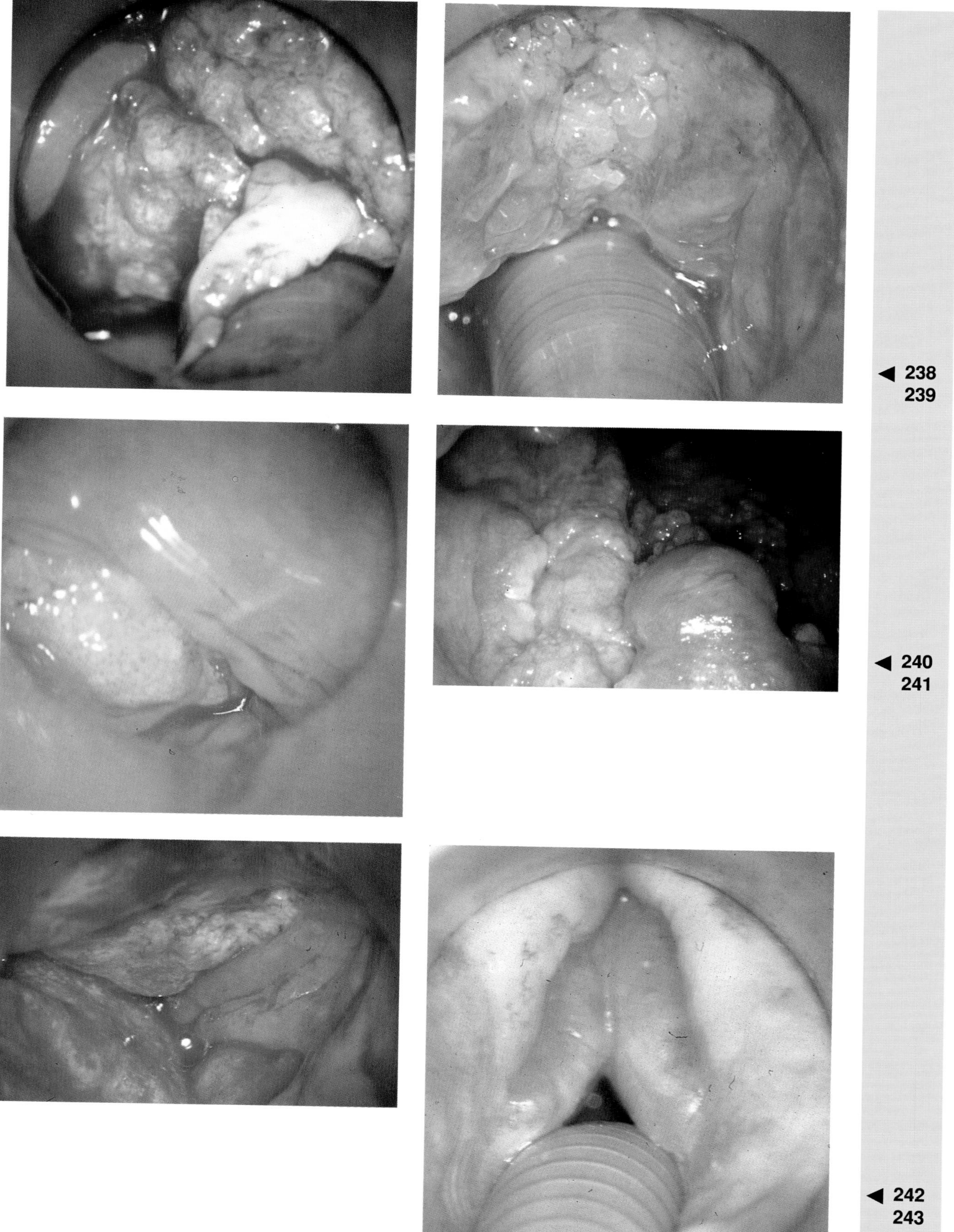

◀ 238
239

◀ 240
241

◀ 242
243

An endoscopic resection should only be carried out if a good view can be obtained with the laryngoscope of the entire tumor and the surrounding area. Tumors that can only be inspected badly or only with a narrow laryngoscope must be treated by an external procedure, which always allows tidy excision in one piece. In principle I only treat carcinomas or carcinoma-in-situ by the endoscopic method if the vocal cords are freely mobile. The tumor should not extend more than 5 mm into the infraglottic region; posteriorly the cartilaginous part of the glottis should not be invaded, and laterally the tumor should not extend into the ventricle. On the other hand, extension across the anterior commissure is not a contraindication to endoscopic resection. Also, superficially spreading carcinomas extending over a large area of both vocal cords can be resected endoscopically, if necessary, at several sittings.

I do not continue with an endoscopic procedure if deeper invasion of the vocal cord musculature is revealed by palpation or by resection. Free mobility of the vocal cords alone is not a certain criterion that the tumor is still superficial. Tumors that have infiltrated more deeply or that have limited the mobility of the vocal cords are not considered for endoscopic resection. It is true that an extensive endoscopic resection, including removal of the entire musculature down to the thyroid perichondrium and large parts of the vestibular folds or the arytenoid cartilage, is technically possible, but I have seen cases with a larynx reduced to an inert scarred tube, and the patient aphonic.

Endoscopic resection of large tumors offers no advantage, because the operation is carried out tangentially under progressively worsening vision in the lateral segment of the laryngeal soft tissues. The remaining defect leads inevitably to extensive scarring, glottic insufficiency, and a poor voice. In such cases an external approach has the advantage of offering a good view of the entire operative field and the ability to adjust the extent of the resection accurately to the size of the tumor. Furthermore, an external operation has the advantage of allowing immediate functional reconstruction of the glottis in a way that is not technically possible by endoscopy.

A previous biopsy carried out elsewhere may make an endoscopic procedure extremely difficult if not impossible, even for cases where it would have originally been suitable, because the boundaries of the tumor can no longer be clearly defined. I carry out about 90% of endoscopic resections of premalignant lesions and carcinomas of the vocal cord in one sitting without a previous biopsy. The microlaryngoscopic appearance of the carcinoma is so characteristic that the biopsy and the definitive treatment can usually be combined. If microscopic examination shows that the lesion was a benign keratoma or a senile papilloma, further surgery is unnecessary.

The resection begins by circumscribing the tumor laterally or inferiorly, followed by dissection from the underlying layer, steering clear of the vocal ligament. Dissection is carried more deeply into the vocal cord if the tumor cannot be elevated smoothly from the muscle of if hard areas are found in the muscle. If it turns out that the tumor is infiltrating more deeply, the endoscopic approach is abandoned in favor of an external access.[33]

It is certainly possible to resect a tumor extending across the anterior commissure in one piece, but the functional results are often better if the smaller half of the tumor is left behind and resected later. I usually carry out the operation in one sitting for minimal contralateral spread, but in two sittings about 4 weeks apart for more extensive disease. Postoperative web formations of the anterior commissure are surprisingly uncommon after endoscopic resection. However, the patient must be watched carefully in the postoperative period, and extensive fibrin membranes or granulomas must be removed immediately.

Careful histologic assessment of the specimen is a further essential prerequisite of endoscopic resection of a vocal cord carcinoma and every partial resection (see page 29). If this time-consuming microscopic assessment is not available, partial resection should not be carried out and the patient should be treated by irradiation.

If histologic examination shows that the tumor has not been completely removed, immediate reoperation is preferable. Sometimes it is not possible to be sure, even with careful histologic analysis, whether the line of section lies exactly at the edge of the tumor or whether tumor remains beyond the margin. The question should not be determined by a wait and see policy but by immediate reoperation. If histologic examination shows a superficial finger of tumor, this can often be removed by endoscopy. However, if there is uncertainty about the deep margin within the vocal cord muscles, a cordectomy through an external laryngotomy is preferred.

In a personal series of 106 patients treated by endoscopy for a small vocal cord carcinoma or a carcinoma-in-situ between 1979 and 1990, not a single patient has lost his life, his larynx, or his voice. Two patients have required radiotherapy to treat recurrences. Four small local recurrences, three of which were located on the contralateral cord, were all dealt with by endoscopy.

The outcome in these cases is just as good as radiotherapy with respect to voice, but much better with respect to healing. However, these results can only be achieved by very careful selection. The good results of endolaryngeal microsurgical resection of small vocal cord carcinomas are achieved with minimal time, cost, and trauma.

c. The Larynx After Irradiation (Figures 243–253)

Assessment of the effect of irradiation is often very difficult due to inflammatory changes, edema, swelling, and fibrin membranes. We carry out microlaryngoscopy as a routine 6–8 weeks after the radiotherapy, and then at 6 months and 1 year.[28] During this period of time a series of changes comes over the tumor and the larynx, which the laryngologist must recognize and be able to assess.

Radiation Mucositis. The first change to occur during irradiation is radiation mucositis (Figures 243–245) characterized by generalized swelling and redness of the laryngeal epithelium. In more marked cases a tenacious yellowish fibrin membrane forms, which must often be removed mechanically by suction before the mucosa can be assessed. Erythema and edema are very variable and depend, among other things, on radiation techniques such as dose, the type of irradiation, and fractionation. A fibrinous corditis is unusual; it can persist for up to a year and is characterized by thick swelling and a tenacious fibrin membrane on one vocal cord.

Tumor Necrosis. This usually begins after delivery of a dose of 40 to 60 Gy and often persists for 4–8 weeks. Ulcers of varying depth often develop at the site of the tumor, and these can be slow to heal and re-epithelialize. Tumor tissue that can still be recognized 8 weeks after the end of irradiation usually indicates a residual carcinoma that demands a biopsy and further treatment (Figures 246–247).

Persistent swelling or fixation of the vocal cord with no visible tumor can be particularly difficult to assess. Even with microlaryngoscopy, it may often be impossible to decide whether this condition is due to residual tumor, persisting inflammation, or chondroradionecrosis. In such cases a wide-bore needle biopsy is sometimes helpful, although the results may be inconclusive.

Radiation Atrophy of the Epithelium (Figures 247–249). This appears about 3 months after the irradiation, once the mucositis has resolved. The epithelium becomes increasingly thinner, white, and difficult to move over the underlying Reinke's space. Increased tortuous dilated capillaries develop on the vocal cords. In many cases the entire vocal cord appears hard and fibrosed, and this condition can even worsen with time, leading to deterioration of the voice. Whereas the well-known atrophy of the skin of the neck has become unusual since the advent of cobalt irradiation, atrophy of the laryngeal epithelium has become more common.

Chondroradionecrosis may be an early or late complication (Figure 250) characterized by chronic laryngeal edema, pain on movement of the larynx, pain irradiating to the ear, and fistulae either internally or externally to the skin. Sadly, chondroradionecrosis is often associated with residual carcinoma. In some cases it may be possible to open up a fistula and remove sequestrated cartilage by endoscopy.

Irradiation-induced carcinomas can develop many years later within the irradiated field, usually on the vocal cords. Characteristically, the laryngeal mucosa shows radiation atrophy in addition to the new tumor (Figures 251–253). Histologic examination shows that the tumor has again arisen from the superficial squamous epithelium and not from dormant rests of tumor lying deeply within the tissue.[13, 16, 41]

d. Miscellaneous Tumors

In addition to squamous cell carcinoma there are numerous benign and malignant tumors which may arise in the larynx but are so unusual that a laryngologist may see them only a few times or indeed not at all during his working lifetime. A review of these tumors has been published elsewhere[26, 27] and the description here will be limited to some of the better known tumors.

Tumors of the Mucous Glands of the Larynx. The only adenoma or adenocarcinoma of any importance in the larynx is adenoid cystic carcinoma. Most patients are between 40 and 70 years old, and men are more often affected than women. About 80% of these tumors develop between the subglottic surface of the vocal cord and the upper tracheal rings. Adenoid cystic carcinomas of the epiglottis and the vestibular folds are rare. The tumor appears smooth or nodular under an intact mucosa with increased capillaries, and it projects only a little into the laryngeal lumen. These tumors usually lie posteriorly in the laryngotracheal junctional zone and only seldom on the lateral wall of the larynx or trachea. The true extent of the tumor is usually several times greater than the endolaryngeal appearances suggest. Diagnosis can only be made by biopsy.

Pleomorphic adenomas, mucoepidermoid tumors, and other adenomas and adenocarcinomas are extremely unusual and do not have any characteristic appearances.

Fig. 244.

Marked edema of the entire laryngeal soft tissues. Demarcation and necrosis of the tumor covered by fibrin.

Fig. 245.

Appearance after completion of irradiation. The swelling of the vocal cords is resolving. The fibrin membrane persists on the left side, and an ulcer at the site of the tumor can be seen on the right side.

Fig. 246.

Residual carcinoma 1 month after completion of radiotherapy with resolving radiation mucositis.

Fig. 247.

Residual or recurrent tumor appearing within 1 year of completion of radiotherapy, with already established pronounced atrophy of the vocal cord epithelium.

Fig. 248.

Irradiation atrophy of the epithelium, persistence of submucosal edema, and very marked capillary hyperplasia.

Fig. 249.

Pronounced unilateral epithelial atrophy of the vocal cord 10 years after contact irradiation with a radium source.

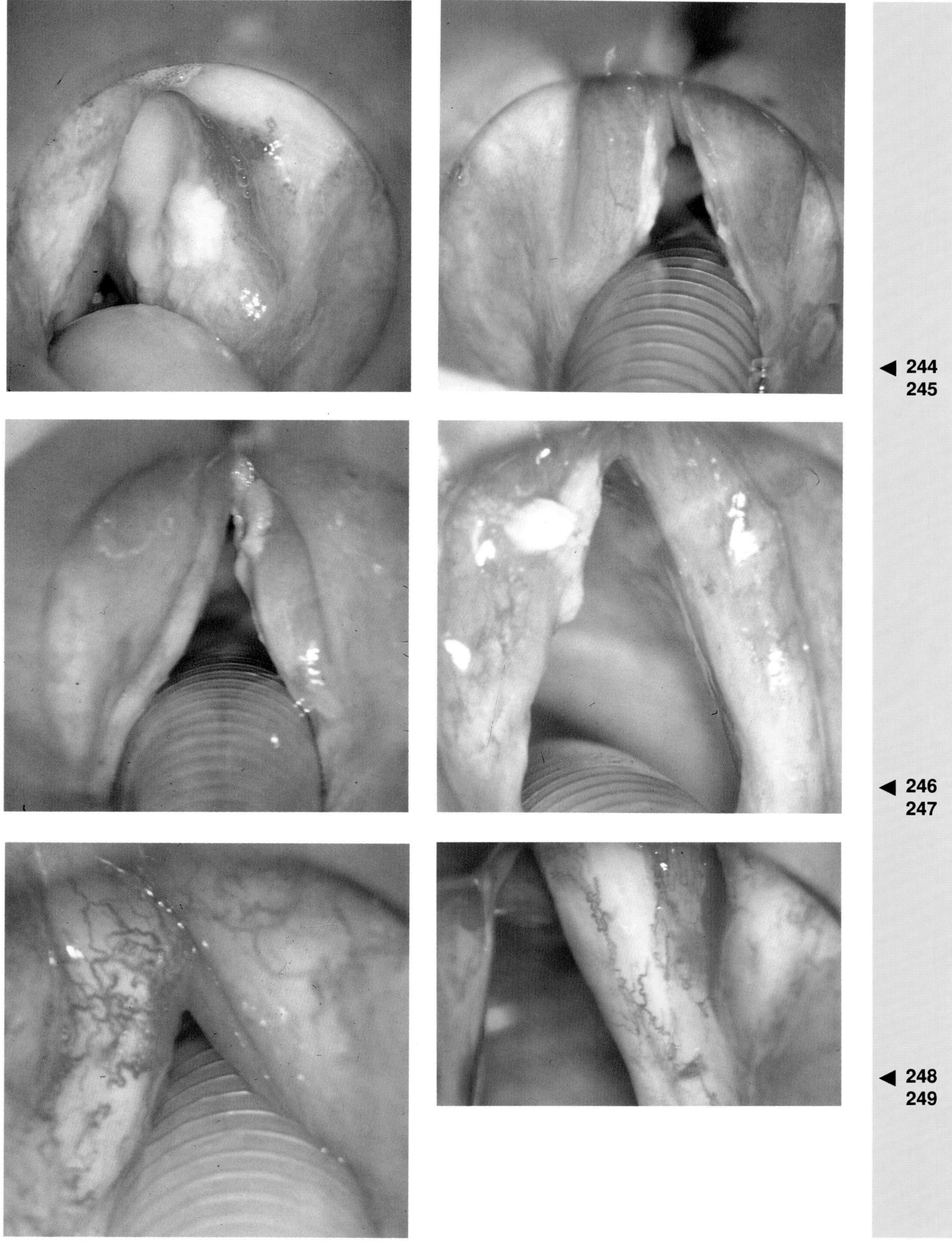

◀ 244
245

◀ 246
247

◀ 248
249

Neuroendocrine tumors: carcinoids of the larynx arise almost exclusively in elderly men, and originate mostly from the aryepiglottic fold or the vestibular fold up to the pharyngo-epiglottic ligament.[26] Microlaryngoscopy shows a red, nodular tumor covered by smooth, intact mucosa, usually with a diameter of 1–2 cm.

Oat cell carcinomas of the larynx are about three times more common in men than women. The men are almost always smokers and 50 to 60 years old. Oat cell carcinomas mainly develop in the subglottic region and at the time of diagnosis have often metastasized to regional lymph nodes and have also produced hematogenous metastases.

Microlaryngoscopy often shows a bilateral, diffuse subglottic swelling, sometimes associated with unilateral or bilateral vocal cord paralysis. The mucosa of the tumor is usually smooth and intact.

Paragangliomas: nonchromaffin paragangliomas (glomus tumors or chemodectomas) of the larynx arise almost exclusively from the superior laryngeal glomus in the posterior part of the vestibular fold (Figure 254). Very occasionally they arise outside the larynx in the space between the thyroid and cricoid cartilages and thereafter invade the larynx secondarily. Most patients are between 50 and 70 years old, and men are slightly more often affected than women. Microlaryngoscopy shows a red, sometimes pulsating tumor covered by a smooth, thin mucosa. At first sight the tumor resembles a hemangioma, and this should be a warning against a hasty biopsy; massive bleeding may follow biopsy of a glomus tumor of the larynx.[26]

Small nonchromaffin paragangliomas can be resected endoscopically, but larger tumors are more suitably dealt with by an external approach. The assessment should include angiography. Malignant types producing multiple skin and scalp metastases are rare (Figure 255).

Fig. 250.

Chondroradionecrosis. The completely necrotic arytenoid cartilage can be seen jutting into a deep defect in the left vocal cord.

Fig. 251.

Carcinoma-in-situ of the right vocal cord, 15 years after thyrotomy and irradiation.

Fig. 252.

Radiation-induced carcinoma of the right vocal cord 8 years after completion of irradiation showing well-established atrophy of the vocal cord epithelium.

Fig. 253.

Radiation-induced carcinoma arising 10 years after radiotherapy for vocal cord carcinoma. Athrophy of the mucosa of the right vocal cord is still clearly recognizable.

Fig. 254.

Small nonchromaffin paraganglioma at the typical site posteriorly in the region of the vestibular and aryepiglottic folds. This tumor was removed endoscopically.

Fig. 255.

Metastasizing paraganglioma in the supraglottic larynx.

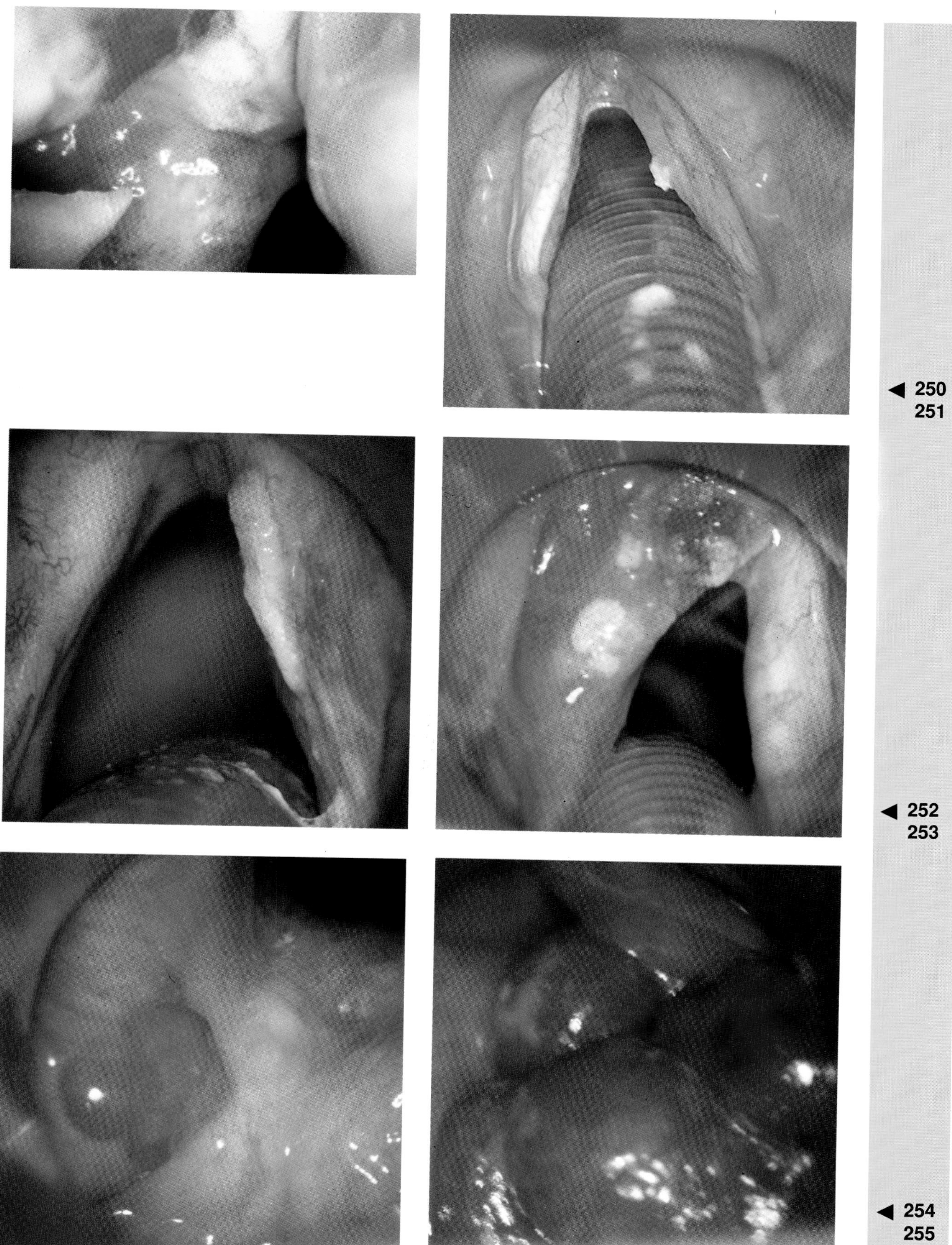

◀ 250
251

◀ 252
253

◀ 254
255

Neurogenic tumors: schwannomas present in the fourth and fifth decades, slightly more often in men than in women, and arise almost exclusively from the aryepiglottic fold in the region of the apex of the arytenoid cartilage (Figure 256). The tumor is smooth and encapsulated; it usually has a pedicle and can therefore easily be removed by the endoscopic route.

Neurofibromas of the larynx occur almost exclusively in neurofibromatosis, usually presenting in children or adolescents. Multiple neurofibromas can lead to fixation of the arytenoid (Figure 257).

About 50% of all granular cell tumors arise in the head and neck, principally in the tongue, but about 10% are found in the larynx.[45] The patients are usually middle aged, and there is no sex predilection. Laryngeal granular cell tumors arise almost exclusively on the vocal cords, particularly in the posterior part at the junction with the arytenoid cartilage (Figure 258). The tumor may lie more deeply in the muscle and then is characterized only by a diffuse swelling of one vocal cord. Other cases demonstrate solid nodular or polypoid tumors greyish-red in color. These tumors can usually be removed by endoscopy. They extend deeply into the muscle and can only be delineated with difficulty, but recurrences are very unusual.

Lymphomas: non-Hodgkin's and Hodgkin's lymphomas are occasionally found in the larynx, usually associated with generalized disease. Extramedullary plasmacytomas may also be found in the larynx, most often in the supraglottic area and more rarely in the subglottic space (Figures 259, 260).

The patients are usually between the ages of 40 and 70 years, and men are affected three times more commonly than women. The tumors are nodular and pedicled, but sometimes form only a diffuse swelling. They are red or yellowish-red in color, and the overlying mucosa is usually smooth and intact with pronounced capillaries. These tumors are seldom larger than 1.5 cm in size.

Small plasmacytomas can be resected endoscopically. The tumors have no sharp boundaries with the deeper tissues and can also destroy part of the laryngeal skeleton. Endoscopic resection should be followed by irradiation.

Fig. 256.

Typical schwannoma arising from the aryepiglottic fold on a pedicle.

Fig. 257.

Bilateral neurofibromas arising from the region of the vocal process.

Fig. 258.

Granular cell tumor arising at the typical site from the posterior part of the left vocal cord.

Fig. 259.

Plasmacytoma of the anterior wall of the subglottis.

Fig. 260.

Extenisve solitary soft tissue plasmacytoma in the supraglottic part of the larynx.

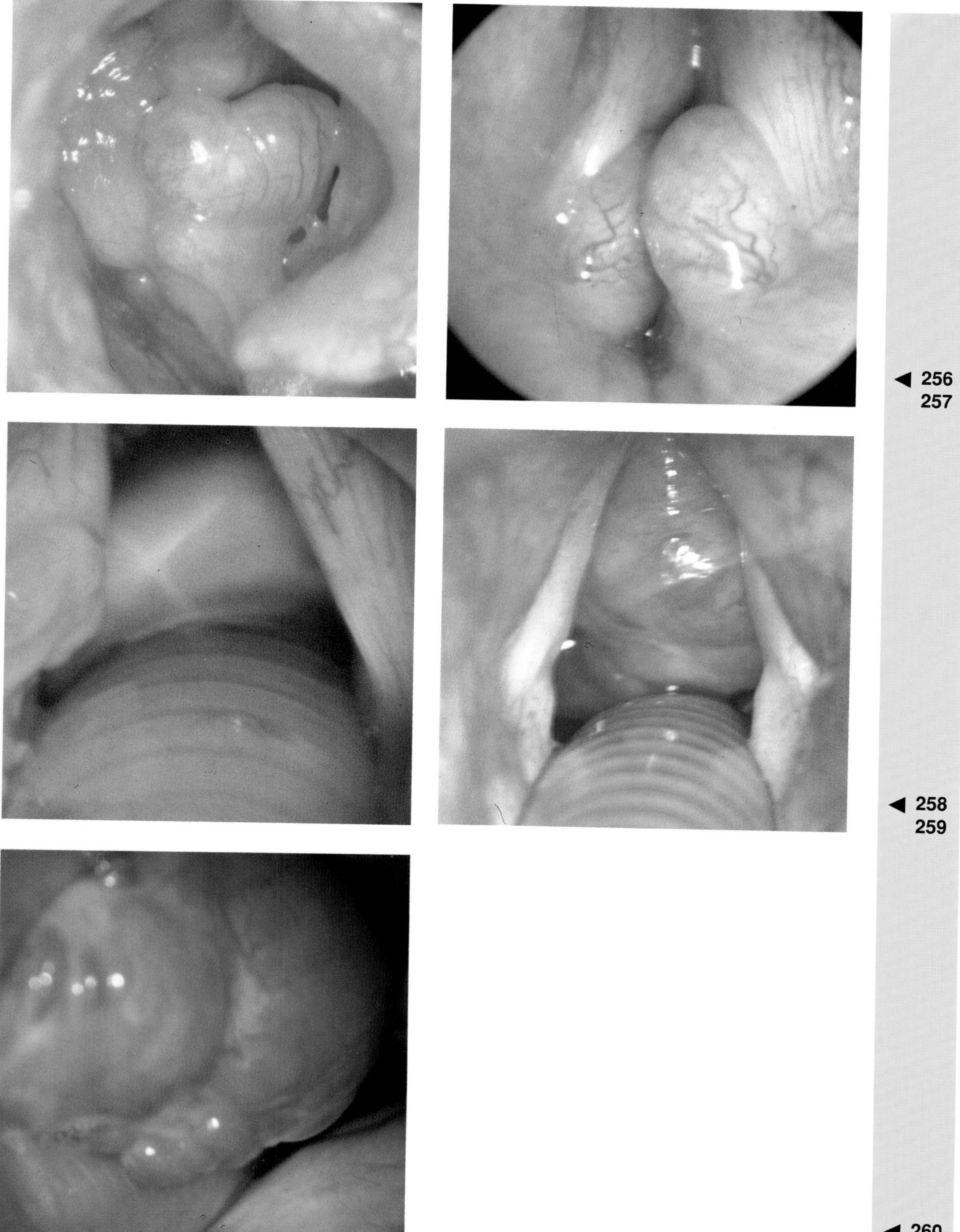

◀ 256
257

◀ 258
259

◀ 260

Wegener's granuloma usually affects the supraglottic part of the larynx, presenting as an ulcer lined by a viscous membrane and affecting the vestibular fold or the arytenoid region (Figures 261, 262). If this is the sole lesion, the diagnosis may be difficult to make from a biopsy.

Vascular tumors: capillary hemangiomas of infants are usually seen in the first weeks or months of life and present with increasing stridor. In about 50% of cases a capillary hemangioma is found on the skin, making diagnosis easier. Microlaryngoscopy shows that the tumor almost always lies in the subglottic space and that the main part of the mass arises from the posterior wall of the larynx. The tumor is bluish-red in appearance, easily compressible, and covered by delicate mucosa. Biopsy is contraindicated because of the danger of bleeding.

The preferred treatment is long-term tracheostomy until the tumor undergoes spontaneous resolution, usually at the age of 2 or 3 years.[52]

Aggressive treatment using the laser, irradiation, or external surgery usually demands tracheotomy and is not indicated.[52]

Cavernous hemangiomas are occasionally found in the supraglottic region or the hypopharynx. Removal by endoscopy is usually attended by surprisingly little bleeding, so that most of these tumors can be removed by this method (Figures 263, 264).

Miscellaneous sarcomas: fibrosarcomas of the vocal cords, malignant histiocytoma, leiomyosarcoma and rhabdomyosarcoma, liposarcoma, and synovioma are very rare and have no characteristic appearance. Most synoviomas arise in the hypopharynx.

Tumors of the laryngeal skeleton: the only tumor of any frequency is chondrosarcoma. It almost always arises from the cricoid plate of the arytenoid region and narrows the laryngeal aditus, so that intubation is no longer possible (Figure 265). The tumor is bony hard to palpation, and a robust punch is often needed to obtain enough tissue for biopsy. The extent of the tumor can be defined accurately by radiography.

Fig. 261.

Wegener's granuloma extensively destroying the right vestibular fold and arytenoid region.

Fig. 262.

Wegener's granuloma showing a deep ulcer on the right vestibular fold and aryepiglottic region.

Fig. 263.

Cavernous hemangioma of the right vestibular fold.

Fig. 264.

Extensive cavernous hemangioma of both piriform fossae and the posterior laryngeal wall.

Fig. 265.

Large chondroma of the cricoid cartilage extending into the hypopharynx. A food remnant can be seen in the right piriform fossa.

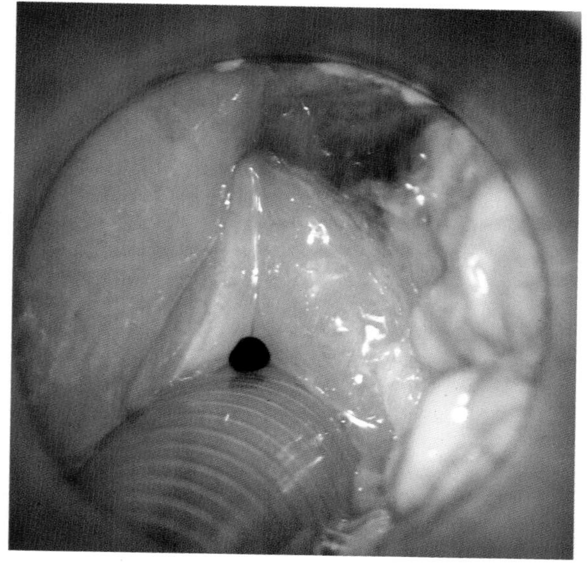

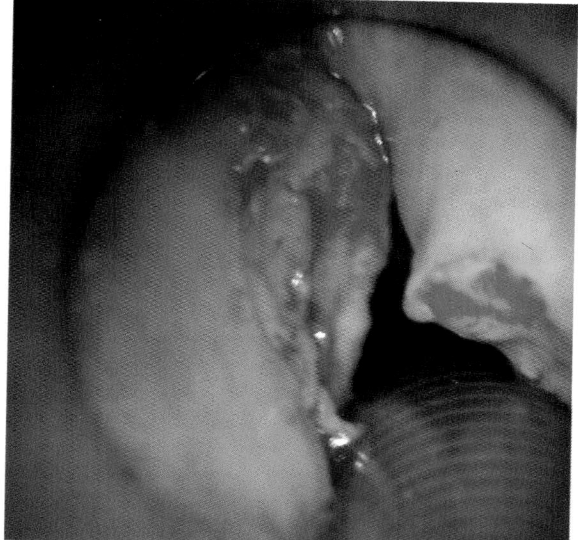

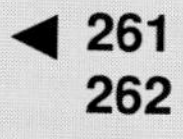

◀ 261
262

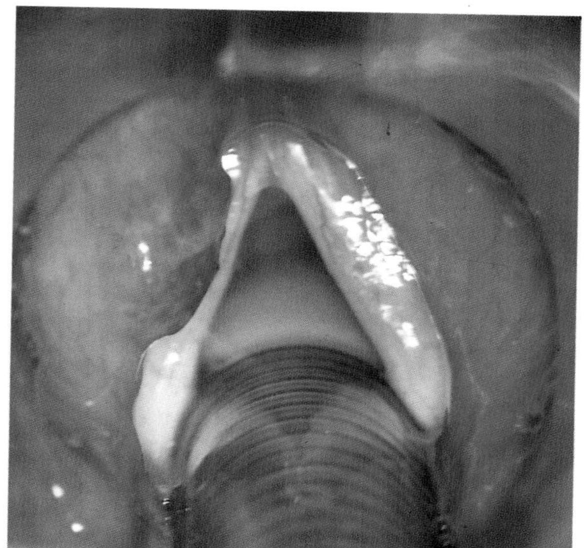

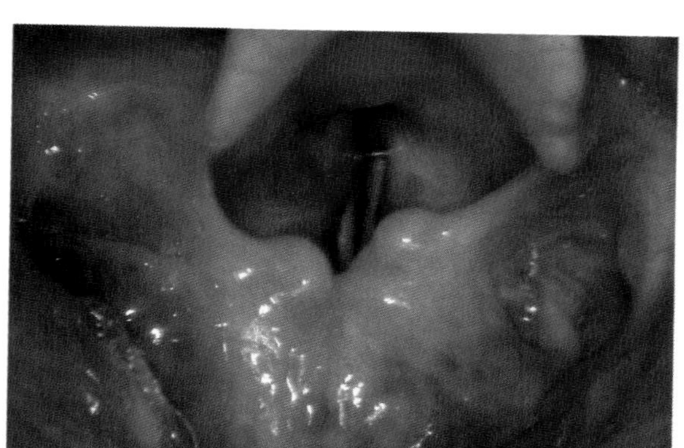

◀ 263
264

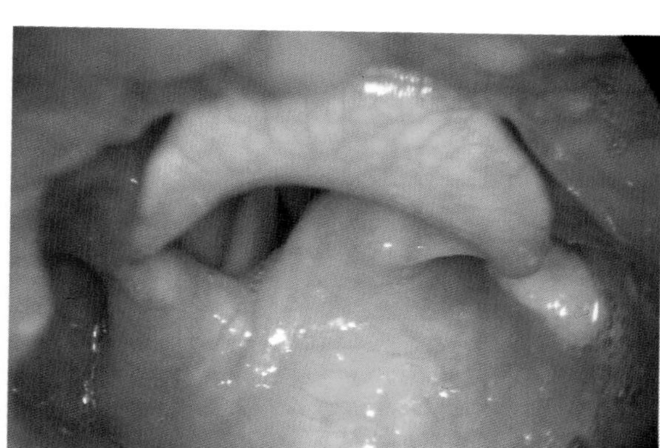

◀ 265

References

1. Abitbol J. Vocal cord hemorrhages in voice professionals. J of Voice 1988; 2: 261–266.
2. Albanese S, Kleinsasser O. Kongenitale Zysten des Larynx. Laryng Rhinol Otol 1988; 67: 282–285.
3. Bouchayer M, Cornut G. Le sulcus glottidis. Essai de clarification nosologique et étio-pathogénique. Revue de Laryngol 1987, Suppl: 391–393.
4. Bouchayer M, Cornut G, Witzig E, Loire R, Roch J. Epidermoid cysts, sulci, and mucosal bridges of the true vocal cord. Laryngoscope 1985; 95: 1087–1094.
5. Cornut G, Bouchayer M. Etudes sur la voix. Bilan de quinze années entre phoniatre et phonochirurgien. Bull Audio Phonat. Ann Sci Univ Franche 1988; Comté IV: 7–50.
6. Dedo HH, Jackler RK. Laryngeal papilloma. Results of treatment with the CO_2 laser and podophyllum. Ann of Otol 1982; 91: 425–430.
7. Demard F. Laryngitis et états précancéreux. Rev de Laryng 1987; Suppl: 405–409.
8. Feder RJ. Varix of the vocal cord in the professional voice user. Otolaryngol Head Neck Surg 1983; 91: 435–440.
9. Feder RJ, Mitchell MF. Hyperfunctional, hyperacidic, and intubation granulomas. Arch of Otolaryngol 1984; 110: 582–584.
10. Frenzel H, Kleinsasser O, Hort W. Licht- und elektronenmikroskopische Untersuchungen an Stimmlippen des Menschen. Virchows Archiv (Path Anat) 1980; 389: 189–204.
11. Fuchs B. Zur Pathogenese und Klinik des Reinke-Ödems. Langzeitstudie HNO (Berlin) 1989; 37: 490–495.
12. Glanz H, Kimmich T, Eichhorn Th, Kleinsasser O. Behandlungsergebnisse bei 584 Kehlkopfcarcinomen an der Hals-Nasen-Ohrenklinik der Universität Marburg. HNO (Berlin) 1989; 37: 1–10.
13. Glanz H, Kleinsasser O. Radiogene Zweitcarcinome des Larynx. HNO (Berlin) 1976; 24: 48–59.
14. Glanz H, Kleinsasser O. Chronische Laryngitis und Carcinom. Arch Oto-Rhino-Laryngol 1976; 212: 57–75.
15. Glanz H, Kleinsasser O. Verrucous carcinoma of the larynx – a misnomer. Arch Oto-Rhino-Laryngol 1987; 244: 108–111.
16. Glanz H. Late recurrence or radiation induced cancer of the larynx. Clin Otolaryngol 1979; 1: 123–129.
17. Hirano M. Objective evaluation of the human voice: clinical aspects. Fol phoniatr 1989; 41: 89–144.
18. Hirano M, Kurita S. Histologic structure of the vocal fold and its normal and pathological variations. In: Kirchner JA (ed). Vocal fold histopathology. 1986; San Diego: College Hill Press 17–24.
19. Jako GJ. Microsurgery of the larynx with the CO_2-laser. Arch Otolaryngol 1979; 3: 1–20.
20. Kambic V, Radsel Z, Zargi M, Acko M. Vocal cord polyps: incidence, histology and pathogenesis. J Laryngol Otol 1981; 95: 609–618.
21. Kitzing P. Stroboscopy – a pertinent laryngological examination. J of Otolaryngol 1985; 14: 151–157.
22. Kleinsasser O. Mikrolaryngoskopie and endolaryngeale Mikrochirurgie. HNO (Berlin) 1974; 22: 33–38, 69–83
23. Kleinsasser O. Mikrolaryngoskopie und endolaryngeale Mikrochirurgie. 2. Auflage. Stuttgart: Schattauer 1976.
24. Kleinsasser O. Pathogenesis of vocal cord polyps. Ann Otol Rhinol 1982; 91: 378–381.
25. Kleinsasser O. Bemerkungen zur Laser-Chirurgie. Arch Otorhinolaryngol 1987; Suppl 2: 14–16.
26. Kleinsasser O. Tumoren des Larynx und Hypopharynx. Stuttgart: Thieme 1987.
27. Kleinsasser O. Tumors of the larynx and hypopharynx. New York: Thieme Medical Publishers, 1988.
28. Kleinsasser O, Friedmann G. Endoskopische Kontrolle des Bestrahlungsverlaufes bei Stimmlippenkarzinomen. Endoscopy 1970; 2: 145–148.
29. Kleinsasser O, Glanz H. Sarkomähnliche Gewebsbilder in Larynxkarzinomen: Laryngol Rhinol Otol 1979; 57: 225–234.
30. Kleinsasser O, Glanz H. Spontane Kanzerisierung nicht bestrahlter juveniler Larynxpapillome. Laryngol Rhinol Otol 1979; 58: 481–488.
31. Kleinsasser O, Glanz H. Microcarcinoma and microinvasive carcinoma of the vocal cords. Clinics in Oncol 1982; 1: 479–487.
32. Kleinsasser O, Glanz H. Histologisch kontrollierte Tumorchirurgie. HNO (Berlin) 1984; 32: 234–236.
33. Kleinsasser O, Glanz H, Kimmich T. Endoskopische Chirurgie bei Stimmlippenkarzinomen. HNO (Berlin) 1988; 36: 412–416.
34. Kleinsasser O, Kruse E, Schönhärl E. Taschenfaltenhyperplasien des Kehlkopfes (Pathogenese und Behandlung). HNO (Berlin) 1975; 23: 29–34.
35. Kleinsasser O, Schroeder HG, Glanz H. Medianverlagerung gelähmter Stimmlippen mittels Knorpelspanimplantation und Türflügelthyreoplastik. HNO (Berlin) 1982; 30: 275–279.
36. Kleinsasser O, Nolte E. Endolaryngeale Arytaenoidektomie und submuköse partielle Chordektomie bei bilateralen Stimmlippenlähmungen. Laryngol Rhinol Otol 1981; 60: 397–401.
37. von Leden H. Microlaryngoscopy: a historical vignette. J of Voice 1988; 1: 341–346.
38. von Leden H. Legal pitfals in laryngology. J of Voice 1988; 2: 330–333.
39. Lehmann W, Pampurik J, Guyot JPH. Laryngeal pathologies observed in microlaryngoscopy. ORL 1989; 51: 206–215.
40. Lehmann W, Pinoux JM, Widmann JJ. Larynx, microlaryngoscopie et histopathologie. Cadempino: Inpharzam Medical Publications 1981.
41. Martin G, Glanz H, Kleinsasser O. Ionisierende Strahlen und Kehlkopfkrebse. Laryngol Rhinol Otol 1979; 58: 187–195.
42. Michaels L. Pathology of the larynx. Berlin: Springer 1984.
43. Monday LA, Cornut G, Bouchayer M, Roch JB. Epidermoid cysts of the vocal cords. Ann Otol Rhinol Laryngol 1983; 124–127.
44. Nielsen VM, Højslet PE, Karlsmose M. Surgical treatment of Reinke's oedema. J Laryngol Otol 1986; 100: 187–190.
45. Nolte E, Kleinsasser O. Granularzelltumoren des Kehlkopfes. HNO (Berlin) 1982; 30: 333–339.
46. Nolte E, Kleinsasser O. Amyloidablagerungen im Kehlkopf. Laryngol Rhinol Otol 1984. 63: 251–254.
47. Otte TH, Kleinsasser O. Endotracheale Dystopien von Schilddrüsengewebe. HNO (Berlin) 1984; 32: 213–216.
48. Reling J. Industrielle Endoskopie: Systeme Komponenten Anwendung. Bibliothek d. Technik, Vol 25. Landsberg: Verlag Moderne Industrie 1988.
49. Remenar E, Élö J, Frint T. The morphological basis for development of Reinke's oedema. Acta Otolaryngol 1984; 97: 169–176.
50. Sawashima M, Hirose H. New laryngoscopic technique by use of fiber optics. J Acoust Soc. Am 1968; 43: 168–169.
51. Schönhärl E. Die Stroboskopie in der praktischen Laryngologie. Stuttgart: G. Thieme 1960.

52. Sebastian B, Kleinsasser O. Zur Behandlung der Kehlkopfhämangiome bei Kindern. Laryngol Rhinol Otol 1984; 63: 403–407.
53. Sebastian B, Kleinsasser O. Die Sarkoidose des Kehlkopfes. Laryngol Rhinol Otol 1985; 64: 622–626.
54. Sebastian B, Kleinsasser O. Einbruch von Schilddrüsentumoren in Larynx und Trachea. Laryngol Rhinol Otol 1985; 64: 128–132.
55. Sopko J. Klinische Laryngologie. Basel: Inpharzam Med Publikation 1987.
56. von Stuckrad H, Lakatos I. Über ein neues Lupenlaryngoskop (Epipharyngoskop). Laryngol Rhinol Otol 1975; 54: 336–340.
57. Wahab AM. Microlaryngoscopy in some phoniatric disorders. Thesis El-Mansour Faculty Egypt 1989.
58. Wolters B, Eichhorn Th, Kleinsasser O. Kritische Betrachtungen zur Therapie der juvenilen Kehlkopfpapillome. Laryngol Rhinol Otol 1984; 63: 396–400.
59. Ward PH, Zwitman D, Hanson D, Berci G. Contact ulcers and granulomas of the larynx. Otol Head Neck Surg 1960; 88: 262.
60. Yanagisawa E., Casuccio JR, Suzuki M. Video laryngoscopy using a rigid telescope and video home system color camera. Ann Otol Rhinol 1981;90: 346–350.

Conclusion

The third edition of this book is dedicated to an attempt to summarize the continued development of microlaryngoscopy and endolaryngeal microsurgery. These diagnostic and therapeutic methods have now found a permanent place worldwide in laryngology, and they have taught us much about the pathogenesis and clinical appearances of the various diseases of the larynx. However, numerous questions remain unanswered; for example, we still do not know the cause of common diseases such as Reinke's edema. Advances will only be made by devoting our attention in the future to the etiology and pathogenesis of laryngeal diseases; only then will we be able to offer treatment based on the cause of the disease rather than the current mechanistic surgical treatment of symptoms.

Index